# Evidence Report

## Number 75

# Screening for Depression in Adults and Older Adults in Primary Care: An Updated Systematic Review

**Prepared for:**
Agency for Health Care Research and Quality
U.S. Department of Health and Human Services
540 Gaither Road
Rockville, MD 20850
www.ahrq.gov
Contract No. 290-02-0024, Task Order Number 1

**Prepared by:**
Oregon Evidence-based Practice Center
Kaiser Permanente Center for Health Research
3800 North Interstate Avenue
Portland, OR 97227

**Investigators:**
Elizabeth A. O'Connor, PhD
Evelyn P. Whitlock, MD, MPH
Bradley Gaynes, MD, MPH (UNC School of Medicine; Department of Psychiatry)
Tracy L. Beil, MS

**AHRQ Publication No. 10-05143-EF-1**

**December 2009**

This report is based on research conducted by the Oregon Evidence-based Practice Center (EPC) under contract to the Agency for Healthcare Research and Quality (AHRQ), Rockville, MD (Contract No. 290-02-0024). The investigators involved have declared no conflicts of interest with objectively conducting this research. The findings and conclusions in this document are those of the author(s), who are responsible for its content, and do not necessarily represent the views of AHRQ. No statement in this report should be construed as an official position of AHRQ or of the U.S. Department of Health and Human Services.

The information in this report is intended to help clinicians, employers, policymakers, and others make informed decisions about the provision of health care services. This report is intended as a reference and not as a substitute for clinical judgment.

This report may be used, in whole or in part, as the basis for the development of clinical practice guidelines and other quality enhancement tools, or as a basis for reimbursement and coverage policies. AHRQ or U.S. Department of Health and Human Services endorsement of such derivative products may not be stated or implied.

**Suggested Citation:** O'Connor EA, Whitlock EP, Gaynes B, Beil TL. Screening for Depression in Adults and Older Adults in Primary Care: An Updated Systematic Review. Evidence Synthesis No. 75. AHRQ Publication No. 10-05143-EF-1. Rockville, Maryland: Agency for Healthcare Research and Quality, December 2009.

# Structured Abstract

**Background:** Depression causes significant suffering and is commonly seen in primary care. Because primary care providers sometimes fail to identify patients as depressed, systematic screening programs in primary care may be of use in improving outcomes in depressed patients. Depression screening is predicated on the notion that identification will allow effective treatments to be delivered and that the benefits of treatment will outweigh the harms. Treatment efficacy of antidepressants and psychotherapy in general adult populations was established in a previous United States Preventive Services Task Force (USPSFT) review on depression screening, but treatment in older adults was not examined specifically. Additionally, harms of screening and treatment were not previously examined in detail.

**Purpose:** This evidence report updates the evidence for the benefits and harms of screening primary care patients for depression in order to initiate or modify treatment aimed at providing relief from depression.

**Data sources:** We developed an analytic framework and five key questions to represent the logical evidence connecting primary care screening to improved health outcomes, including remission from depression. We searched Medline, Cochrane Central Registry of Controlled Trials, and PsycINFO from 1998 to December 2007, and Cochrane Database of Systematic Reviews from 1998 – October 2006 (with updates through December 2007). Separate literature search strategies were developed for harms of screening and harms of treatment. We also considered all trials included in the previous systematic review for the USPSTF and a recent Cochrane review on depression screening in primary care, contacted experts, and checked bibliographies from non-systematic reviews and other studies. We examined 4088 abstracts and 412 full-text articles.

**Study Selection:** For all key questions, we considered evidence from studies published in English that were conducted in the United States or other similarly developed countries and met design-specific USPSTF quality standards. We included fair-to-good quality randomized clinical trials (RCTs) or controlled clinical trials (CCTs) that evaluated screening for depression in primary care settings if the screening and related interventions involved general adult primary care populations and if the control group was either unscreened or the results of the screening were not used in the care of the patient. We found no trials or studies addressing harms of screening. We included good-quality meta-analyses that examined depression treatment efficacy in older adults. We included fair-to-good quality systematic reviews, meta-analyses, and large observational studies of serious adverse events and early discontinuation due to adverse effects in adult and older adults.

**Data Extraction:** One reviewer abstracted relevant information from each included article into standardized evidence tables, and a second reviewer checked all elements. Two reviewers graded the quality of each article using USPSTF criteria. Excluded articles are listed in tables, along with the primary reason(s) for exclusion.

**Data Synthesis:** Programs that include depression screening and staff that assist the primary care clinician by providing some direct depression care (such as care support or coordination, case management, or mental health treatment) can increase depression response and remission over usual care. However, it is unclear whether screening is a necessary component of these programs. Depression screening programs that do not provide depression care supports other than those targeted at improving the effectiveness of the primary care provider's depression treatment (without additional staff involvement) are unlikely to be effective. Antidepressants and psychotherapy are effective in treating depression in older adults, with odds of remission about twice those seen in placebo or other non-active control conditions. The most current evidence on risk of completed suicide deaths does not demonstrate a clear and uniform effect of second-generation antidepressants compared with placebo; rather, data are consistent with no effect, mild protection or some increased risk. Some meta-analyses suggest an increase in suicidal behaviors in young adults (aged 18-29 years) on antidepressants, particularly those with major depressive disorder and those taking paroxetine. In contrast, older adults have a reduced risk of suicidal behaviors during antidepressant treatment.

**Conclusions:** Screening programs without staff-assisted depression care supports are unlikely to improve depression outcomes, although depression treatment can be effective in adults of all ages. Close monitoring of all adult patients initiating antidepressant treatment, particularly those under age 30, is important both for safety reasons and to ensure optimal treatment response.

# Table of Contents

## Appendices

Appendix A. Current practice details
Appendix B. USPSTF Hierarchy of research design and quality rating criteria
Appendix C. Inclusion and exclusion criteria for key questions
Appendix D. Detailed methods
Appendix D Figure 1. Search results and article flow
Appendix D Table 1. Search strategies
Appendix D Figure 2. Screening intervention approaches
Appendix E. Previous adult depression reviews
Appendix F Table 1. Meta-analysis decision factors
Appendix G Table 1. Evidence table of screening trials-KQ1 and KQ1a.
Appendix G Table 2. Evidence table for depression treatment of older adults.
Appendix G Table 3. Summary of rates of suicide and related behavior or ideation.
Appendix G Table 4. Evidence table of systematic evidence reviews and meta-analyses of suicide risk related to SSRIs.
Appendix G Table 5. Evidence table of cohort studies of suicide risk with SSRIs.
Appendix G Table 6. Evidence table of studies of discontinuation of SSRIs.
Appendix G Table 7. Studies excluded from the review.
Appendix G Table 8. Cohort study details
Appendix G Table 9. FDA report

# Chapter 1. Introduction

## Scope and Purpose

We conducted this systematic review to aid the United States Preventive Services Task Force (USPSTF) in updating its 2002 recommendation for adult depression screening in primary care. We focused on gaps in evidence identified by the previous review[1] and on integrating relevant research published in the interim. Questions that the USPSTF judged to have strong, coherent evidence in the previous review are not re-addressed here. Specifically, we did not update evidence regarding the accuracy of screening instruments for identifying depressed adults and older adults in primary care, nor treatment of adult depression with antidepressants or psychotherapy. We updated direct evidence that primary care depression screening programs improve health outcomes and examined evidence for the efficacy of depression treatment in older adults and evidence for the harms of screening and adverse events from antidepressant treatment in adults and older adults.

## Condition Definition

The term "depression" is not a specific term for a single diagnostic condition. Depressive disorders generally consist of major depressive disorder (MDD), dysthymia, and minor depression, but not other conditions that include depressive features, such as bipolar disorder. The American Psychiatric Association[2] specifies diagnostic criteria for the different depressive disorders, each of which requires a minimum number of symptoms to be present and significant distress or impairment (Table 1). MDD is the most serious diagnosis, and is given to a person who meets criteria for major depressive disorder without manic or hypomanic features or a psychotic disorder. Dysthymia is similar to MDD but is generally longer-lasting and less severe. A variety of terms are used for people with depressive symptoms but whose depression does not meet criteria for MDD or dysthymia, such as subthreshold depression, subsyndromal depression, and minor depression. Some studies use the DSM-IV definition of minor depression (developed for research rather than clinical purposes), but many define these patients idiosyncratically so that it is very difficult to compare rates across studies.

## Prevalence and Burden of Disease/Illness

Depressive disorders are common in community and primary care patients. The estimated lifetime prevalence of MDD is approximately 13.2 percent, with a 12-month prevalence of 5 to 7 percent in community-dwelling adults.[3-5] Prevalence Estimates in community-dwelling older adults are much lower (from 1 to 5 percent,[6] with an average of 1.8 percent).[7] A different study found that approximately one to 2.5 percent of older adults are likely to experience a first episode of depression over the course of one year.[8] In primary care settings, the prevalence of MDD ranges from 5 to 13 percent[9-12] in adults and from 6 to 9 percent in older adults.[13,14] For MDD patients receiving treatment in primary care settings, depressive symptoms and severity are equivalent to that seen in MDD patients treated in psychiatric settings; of note, approximately 43 percent of such primary care patients report suicidal ideation within the prior week.[15,16]

Considering other depressive disorders (e.g., dysthymia, and subthreshold depressive disorders) increases the prevalence. Twelve-month prevalence of dysthymia is estimated at 1.5 to 1.6 percent[3,5] in community-dwelling younger (aged 18 to 54) and older (aged ≥ 55) adults.[5] Dysthymia in primary care settings is estimated from 2 to 4 percent.[17] It is difficult to reliably estimate the prevalence of subthreshold disorders in the US due to the wide range of definitions used. In primary care settings, prevalence of broadly defined subthreshold disorders is about 9 percent in adults[18] and 10 percent in older adults.

Depression has been ranked as a leading cause of Years of Life Lived with a Disability (YLD) for persons 15 years and older[19] and the third leading cause of loss in quality-adjusted life years (QALY) in older adults.[20] In addition to its impact on the depressed person, depression is often associated with a drastic loss of productivity at work and home[21,22] and impairment in relationships and social functioning.[21] Depression in parents is associated with behavioral and emotional difficulties in their children.[23-25] Depression may increase the risk of physical disability,[26-29] medical conditions (such as coronary heart disease and diabetes mellitus),[30,31] other mental health conditions, and mortality.[30-34] In one study, the increased mortality seen in depressed older adults was comparable to that seen in patients with emphysema or heart disease.[33] Depression is also a major risk factor for suicide. Suicide mortality among patients treated for depression is estimated at 59 per 100,000 among an insured population.[35]

Depression's economic burden is substantial and includes individual costs (suffering, treatment side effects, possible suicide, health care and medication fees, work disability, and lost earnings); costs to family and friends (informal care-giving, time off work, career burden); employer costs (contributions to treatment and care, reduced productivity); and costs to society (costs of mental health and general medical care, reduced productivity, and loss of lives).[36] In 2000, combined direct and indirect costs of depression in the US were estimated at 83.1 billion dollars, 31.5 billion in direct costs and the remaining in indirect, mostly workplace costs.[37] A 2006 study of depression costs in Europe indicated that 87 percent of the costs associated with depression were indirect costs, such as losses due sickness-related absence from work.[38] Studies of primary care patients have found that health care costs are higher in depressed patients than non-depressed in many categories, including primary care visits, medical specialty visits, lab tests, pharmacy costs, inpatient medical costs, and mental health visits.[31,39] A 1999 study found that while many high utilizers were depressed, their providers often did not recognize their depression.[40]

# Natural History

Depression is a chronic disease characterized by partial remissions and recurrences in most of those who recover fully.[41] While depression can occur in people of any age,[17,21] the average age of onset is in the mid-twenties.[42] Cumulative Kaplan-Meier curves for age-at-onset show fairly low risk until the early teens, with subsequent risk rising in a roughly linear fashion.[21]

Many of the treated depression cases are managed in primary care; roughly one third to one half of non-elderly adults [21,43] and almost two thirds of older adults[44] who are treated for depression are treated in primary care. Large-scale studies of patients initiating treatment for depression indicate that about half to two-thirds of patients achieve remission within a year,[9,45-47] although remission may require up to 4 adequate treatment trials.[46] Patients seen in primary care with depressive disorders whose depression was not recognized by providers do about as well: 50 to 60 percent of these patients are also likely to recover from their depression.[9,47,48] This may be partially due to the fact that patients with unrecognized depression often have less severe symptomatology and impairment.[9,47,49] With provision of evidence-based treatment, recovery rates for identified depressed patients in primary care are equivalent to similarly depressed patients treated in psychiatric settings.[50]

Lower rates of recovery have been seen in population-based studies of depression in the community. Two large Canadian epidemiological databases were used as a basis for developing a depression prognosis calculator, where rate of recovery is estimated from length of current episode.[51] The calculator[52] estimated the 12-month recovery rate for patients whose depression episodes lasted for 12 weeks to be 27 percent, which is considerably lower than the approximately half to two-thirds of patients reported to recover in treatment settings. However, this rate is similar to 28 to 33 percent rate for a single antidepressant trial in the Sequenced Treatment Alternatives to Relieve Depression (STAR*D) study, a large-scale, community-care based effectiveness study of depression treatment.[53]

Older adults have similar or slightly lower recovery rates than younger adults, possibly due to more frequent medical co-morbidities.[54] A meta-analysis of depression in older adult community and primary care populations found that after 2 years an average of 33 percent of patients were categorized as "well," 21 percent had died, and 33 percent still met criteria for full depression. The remaining participants were described as experiencing partial remission or other mental health disorders, such as dementia.[55] This study did not describe recovery rates specifically in treated populations. Similarly, a naturalistic study reporting on the course of depression in older adult primary care patients found that 39 percent of patients with diagnoses of either major or minor depression were in complete remission one year later under usual care conditions[56] and 25 percent still met full criteria for major or minor depression.

Despite fairly high rates of recovery from a particular episode, depression is highly recurrent. A recent evidence-based NICE guideline noted that at least half of individuals diagnosed with depression will have a recurrence following their first episode of depression.[57] This chance of recurrence increases with subsequent episodes. The STAR*D trial found that about half of patients who achieved remission relapsed during the subsequent year.[46]

## Risk Factors for Depression

Individuals are at risk for depression across their entire adult life span. Consistently identified high-risk groups include: women;[6,21,58] people with other psychiatric disorders, including substance misuse;[6,21,59] people with a family history of depression;[6] people with chronic medical diseases;[60] and people who are unemployed or with lower socio-economic status.[6,21,58,61] While the prevalence of MDD is lower in community-dwelling older adults than in younger adults, significant depressive symptomatology is associated with common life events in older adults, including medical illness, cognitive decline, bereavement, and institutional placement in residential or inpatient settings.[6,62]

## Depression in Older Adults

Although MDD is somewhat less prevalent in older adults, depression is a significant public health issue is this age group. Older adults have the highest risk of suicide of all age groups. According to a 1992 NIH Consensus Development Panel on late-life depression, most of these suicidal patients were experiencing their first MDD episode, which had gone unrecognized and untreated.[63] These patients are highly relevant to primary care clinicians because more than 50 to 75 percent of older adults who commit suicide have seen their medical doctor during the prior month for general medical care, and 39 percent are seen during the week prior to their death.[64]

Depression can be particularly difficult to identify in older patients, and much of the burden of depression diagnosis will fall to primary care providers. Diagnosis is complicated because medical conditions or medications can cause symptoms of depression, such as weight loss or appetite change, psychomotor retardation, loss of energy or fatigue, insomnia or hypersomnia, and difficulty concentrating.

Further, the depressive symptoms of depressed mood and feelings of guilt tend to be less prominent in older depressed patients, whose primary complaints tend to be somatic.[65] Depression in older adults is further complicated by the high levels of co-morbidity with medical conditions, including cancer, cardiovascular disease, neurological disorders, metabolic disturbances, arthritis, and sensory loss.[63,66]

# Interventions and Treatment for Depression

Remission of most or all symptoms is the desired outcome of depression treatment[67,68] and is associated with improved functioning in adults.[69] Improvements in depressed mood may help reduce functional decline in older adults.[70]

Response to treatment is typically defined as a reduction of at least 50 percent in baseline symptom levels. Response without full remission, however, is associated with continuing impairments in psychosocial functioning, productivity, continued disabling symptoms and higher levels of health-care use, and higher rates of relapse, recurrence, and potentially suicide.[53]

Effective depression treatment in adults include pharmacotherapy and psychotherapy, delivered singly or in combination.[71] These treatments are widely available for delivery by, or referral from, primary care providers. In samples limited to primary care patients, pharmacologic treatments, such as selective serotonin reuptake inhibitors (SSRIs) and tricyclic antidepressants (TCAs), are more effective than placebo,[72] with some comparative evidence favoring SSRIs over TCAs.[73-75] The reduced tolerability and increased toxicity in overdose of TCAs and other "first-generation" antidepressants has resulted in the use of SSRIs and other "second-generation" antidepressants for the majority of pharmacologic depression treatment delivered in primary care.[76] By 2000, SSRIs accounted for 65 percent of all antidepressants prescribed in primary care and another 17 percent consisting of non-SSRI "second-generation" antidepressants (see Table 2 for listing and categorization of antidepressants).[77] Indeed, between 1996 and 2001, the number of persons using these newer antidepressants increased from 7.9 million to 15.4 million, while the number using TCAs decreased from 2.3 million to 1.2 million.[78]

Remission rates at 12 to 14 weeks with SSRIs range from 22[79] to 28 percent[53] in naturalistic settings, and 35[80] to 47 percent[81] in research settings. Rates of symptom improvement without full remission are higher (47 to 63 percent).[53,75,79,81] Remission rates for psychotherapy appear to be comparable to antidepressants. A systematic review of three-arm, intent-to-treat trials comparing antidepressants, psychotherapy, and a control condition reported 46 percent remission rate for antidepressants and 46 percent remission rate for psychotherapy after 10 to 16 weeks.[82] Additionally, a 2001 Health Technology Assessment Report[83] showed a 52.5 percent overall remission rate for trials comparing some form of psychotherapy with a control condition.

# Current Practice

## Detection and Treatment of Depression in Primary Care

Current mental health screening rates may be as high as 74 percent in primary care, according to Healthy People 2010 midcourse review,[84] although these estimates aren't specific for depression screening. Once a primary care provider has identified a patient as depressed, almost 90 percent of providers recommend antidepressants, either alone or in combination with psychotherapy.[85,86] Only 25 percent of patients receive follow-up visits meeting Healthcare Effectiveness Data and Information Set

(HEDIS) criteria of three visits within the first 12 weeks,[87] and among those patients who initiate antidepressant use, however, up to 40 to 67 percent discontinue use within 3 months[87-89] in real-world settings. This is considerably higher than discontinuation rates reported in the context of clinical trials, where early treatment discontinuation rates range from 16 to 29 percent.[72,75,90-95,46,96] A further synopsis of recent evidence on depression detection and treatment in primary care can be found in Appendix A.

## Proportion of Depression Cases Missed in Primary Care

Although we found no recent evidence on the proportion of depression cases not detected in current primary care in the US, a study in a staff model health maintenance organization (HMO) in western Washington state in the early 1990's suggests that 30 to 40 percent of cases may be missed by primary care providers.[9] In this study, clinicians recognized 64 percent of patients with MDD, and those not recognized were more likely to have less severe depression and to be younger. Three major sets of evidence-based guidelines for recognition and treatment of depression in the US have been developed since this study was conducted, which may have, at minimum, increased awareness of depression and possibly improved the current depression recognition and treatment practices: Agency for Health Care Policy and Research (currently known as AHRQ),[17,97] Veteran's Health Administration (VA),[98] and the American Psychiatric Association (APA).[99] Thus, current recognition rates may be at least comparable to, or possibly higher than, those published in the 1995 study.

# Rationale for Depression Screening

Mass screening in primary care may help clinicians identify missed depression cases and initiate appropriate treatment. Additionally, screening may help clinicians identify patients earlier in their course of depression. In both of these cases, it is presumed that usual care delivers effective treatment and that treating these patients would improve their depression and alleviate their suffering sooner or more thoroughly than if they had not been screened. Unlike other screening tests, screening all patients for depression, including those previously identified as depressed, may be useful since it might help identify ineffectively treated patients whose treatment needs modification.

# Depression Screening Instruments

The previous USPSTF review[71] found that there are reliable and valid depression screening instruments for adults. Screening instruments generally demonstrated sensitivity of 80 to 90 percent and specificity of 70 to 85 percent. The previous reviewers modeled the probability of MDD after a positive screening test using several sensitivity and specificity estimates in these ranges, and background population depression rates of 5, 10, and 15 percent. They estimated that between 12 percent and 50 percent of those screening positive would meet criteria for MDD, with most estimates falling between 24 and 44 percent. Thus, the majority of patients screening positive will not meet criteria for MDD, though some of these may still benefit from counseling or treatment. Clearly, screening instruments are not sufficient for diagnosing depression, but do indicate the need for more detailed follow-up by a clinician to determine whether the person meets diagnostic criteria for a depressive disorder, to explore other possible causes for depression (such as hypothyroidism or medication or substance use), and assess for co-existing psychiatric disorders.

# Controversies about Depression Screening

Since the previous USPSTF-sponsored review,[71] other reviewers have reached different conclusions about depression screening. Pignone et al. concluded that depression screening in primary care is effective in improving health outcomes, but only in the presence of other systems to ensure accurate diagnosis, treatment, and follow-up among patients screening positive.[71] Other reviewers have concluded that screening does not improve health outcomes,[100] but that care management systems for depressed patients significantly improve rates of depression remission.[101] Commentators on these divergent review results have also been divided.[102,103]

# Previous USPSTF Recommendations

In 2002, the U.S. Preventive Services Task Force (USPSTF) recommended screening adults for depression in clinical practices that have systems in place to assure accurate diagnosis, effective treatment, and follow-up (B recommendation).

The USPSTF concluded the evidence is insufficient to recommend for, or against, routine screening of children or adolescents for depression (I recommendation). Since this recommendation's update is being conducted separately, this report only addresses adults.

# Chapter 2. Methods

## Methods Synopsis

Using the USPSTF's methods[104] (Appendices B-D), we developed an analytic framework (Figure 1) and five key questions (KQ) that focused on the evidence the USPSTF required to update its recommendation. For all questions, disorders of interest were Major Depressive Disorder, Dysthymia, Depression Not Otherwise Specified (including Minor Depression), or "depression" with no further diagnostic specificity. However, we did not include evidence that focused *exclusively* on Dysthymia or Minor Depression. KQ1 examined direct evidence that screening programs for depression among adult and older adult primary care patients reduce morbidity and/or mortality. KQ1a examined the impact of clinician feedback of screening test results (with or without additional care management support) on depression response and remission in screen-detected depressed patients receiving primary care. KQ2 examined the adverse effects of screening for depressive disorders in adults and older adults. We did not re-examine screening test accuracy in adults or older primary care patients as that was adequately established in the prior review.[71] KQ3 examined the effectiveness of antidepressant and/or psychotherapy treatment of older adult depressed patients for improving health outcomes, including depression response and remission. The goal of KQ3 was to answer the focused question of whether there are effective agents for treating depression in older adults, and not on identifying the best treatment or the optimal way to implement the treatment. Therefore, we did not include comparative-effectiveness trials or trials that aimed at improving delivery of known effective treatments. We did not update the effectiveness of depression treatment in adults as that was established in the last review.[71] KQ4 assessed the major adverse effects of antidepressant treatments for depression in adults and older adults, with a focus on second-generation antidepressants (SSRIs in particular) due to the preponderance of use of these in the US.

For all key questions, we searched for systematic reviews, meta-analyses, and evidence-based guidelines on depression screening, treatment, or associated harms in adults and older adults in the Database of Abstracts of Reviews (DARE), MEDLINE, and PsycINFO from 1998 through December 2007, and the Cochrane Database of Systematic Reviews (CDSR) from 1998 through October 2006 (with updates through December 2007). Once we identified relevant reviews in the CDSR, we hand-checked for updates periodically through December, 2007. We also conducted a series of searches corresponding to the key questions and reviewed each search for applicability to the other key questions.

For KQ1 and KQ1a, we searched for RCTs/CCTs of depression screening in primary care to cover the time period since the previous USPSTF review (1998 through December, 2007) in MEDLINE, PsycINFO, and Cochrane Collaboration Registry of Clinical Trials (CCRCT). We further searched Science Citation Index, Social Science Citation Index, Science Direct, highWire Press, and Google Scholar from 2000 to March 2006 for articles referencing the single screening trial from the previous USPSTF review that included a non-screened comparison group.[10] In addition to our searches, we considered all screening-related trials identified from the previous USPSTF review,[71] from a 2005 Cochrane review on depression screening,[100] and from a review on educational and organizational interventions for depression[101] for inclusion. Trials were eligible for KQ1 if they compared screened and unscreened patients. For KQ1a, patients must have been screened for depression and the trial must have used the screening results in the care of the intervention participants and must not have used the screening results in the care of the control participants.

For KQ2, we searched MEDLINE and PsyccINFO from 1998 through December, 2007 for trials discussing harms of screening for depression in primary care settings or in populations generalizable to primary care, without restrictions on study designs. For KQ3 we searched MEDLINE, PsycINFO, and CCRCT for systematic evidence reviews, meta-analyses, and trials of psychotherapy and antidepressant treatment in older adults in two separate searches covering 1998 through December, 2007 for psychotherapy and 2003 through December, 2007 for antidepressants. Because we found good-quality recent meta-analyses, we limited our review to synthesized evidence. We did not restrict KQ3 and KQ4 to trials in primary care settings.

For KQ4, we examined all relevant meta-analyses, trials, and large observational studies from several current systematic reviews and evidence-based guidelines addressing treatment-associated harms.[57,92,105] We focused our review of harms on already synthesized evidence supplemented by large observational studies located through searching MEDLINE from 1988 through December, 2007 for publications that included SSRI terms and terms related to either suicide or discontinuation without restrictions with regard to study design. Inclusion and exclusion criteria specific to each question are detailed in Appendix C and D. For screening program and treatment effectiveness, we focused on depression response, remission, and other health outcomes. For harms, we focused on suicide-related events, serious psychiatric events, serious medical events (for older adults), and discontinuation (overall and due to adverse events) as measures of tolerability.

Two investigators reviewed all abstracts. Articles were evaluated against a set of inclusion/exclusion criteria, including design-specific quality criteria based on the USPSTF methods (Appendix B), supplemented by NICE[106] and Oxman[107] criteria for systematic reviews. All studies excluded for quality reasons were critically appraised by two investigators. Data from included studies were abstracted into evidence tables by one investigator and checked by a second. Most data synthesis was qualitative since we judged that trials were not similar enough to allow quantitative syntheses for KQ1 (see Appendix F for between-study differences in potential confounders). For KQ2, we found no data, and we relied on already synthesized evidence for KQ3 and KQ4.

For KQ4, we abstracted data to calculate absolute event rates for suicide-related events from meta-analyses and systematic reviews, with 95 percent confidence interval (CI) calculated based on a Poisson distribution using the SAS version 8.2 GENMOD procedure with the offset option set at the log of the event rate. Risk differences with 95 percent CI for suicide-related events in patients with MDD (a relatively homogeneous risk group) on active medication were calculated using the RISKDIFF option of the FREQ procedure in SAS 8.2. This procedure uses a normal approximation to the binomial distribution to construct asymptotic confidence intervals. (SAS Version 8.2 for Windows, SAS Institute Inc., Cary, North Carolina)

# USPSTF Involvement

The authors worked with four USPSTF liaisons at key points throughout the review process to develop and refine the analytic framework and key questions, resolve issues around scope and approach, and will work with them to finalize this draft report. Research was funded by the Agency for Healthcare Research and Quality (AHRQ) under a contract to support the work of the USPSTF and AHRQ staff provided oversight throughout the project.

# Chapter 3. Results.

## Key Question 1: Is there direct evidence that screening for depression among adults and older adults in primary care reduces morbidity and/or mortality?

**Summary of findings.** One fair-quality randomized controlled trial of primary care patients identified by the previous systematic review[108] compared screening's impact with a non-screened usual care group (Table 3).[10] Nine hundred sixty-nine patients were randomized, 863 of whom completed a post-visit interview. A subset of the randomized patients from one of the two sites, over-sampling those with depressive symptomatology at baseline, were re-assessed after 3-months.

At follow-up, screened patients who were depressed at baseline were more likely to be in complete remission than unscreened depressed patients ($\leq 1$ symptom of depression in 48 percent of those screened compared to 27 percent of those not screened, $p<0.05$). However, when the entire follow-up sample was considered (not merely those who were depressed at baseline), screened and unscreened samples did not differ in the proportion of patients meeting DSM-III-R criteria for a depressive disorder nor in the average change in number of depression symptoms at follow-up. The study's follow-up procedures may have limited their power to detect group differences and introduced bias. This study was also at risk for intervention contamination because providers saw patients in both study conditions. (See Appendix F Table 1 for key elements of the trial and Appendix G Table 1 for detailed information)

**Study details.** Table 4 lists brief information regarding depression screening and interview instruments described in this and subsequent sections. Williams and colleagues[10] conducted the only study that compared a screened sample to a non-screened sample, which is the optimal comparison for looking at the effects of mass screening. Participants were recruited at two sites: a VA general internal medicine clinic in San Antonio, Texas and a university-affiliated general internal medicine clinic in Washington, DC. Patients were randomized either to usual care, to complete a brief (one item) depression screener, or to complete the Center for Epidemiologic Studies-Depression Scale (CESD) before a scheduled appointment. In both screening groups, the results were placed in the patient's chart on a bright orange form, regardless of whether the screening test was positive or negative. Providers saw both intervention and control participants and therefore contamination is possible. All providers were given a guide for managing depression in primary care and a continuing education session on diagnosing depression. No other depression care support was provided.

After the baseline visit with the provider, research staff attempted to interview all randomized (n=969) participants by phone to determine whether they met DSM-III-R criteria for depression; 863 (89.1 percent) completed the post-visit interview. Three months after the index visit, they attempted to contact 230 participants (26.7 percent, 230/863), which included all patients at one study site who met DSM-III-R criteria for a depressive disorder at the post-visit phone interview (n=101), and a random sample at the same site (n=129) who did not meet criteria for depression, over-sampling those who had depressive symptoms without meeting DSM-III-R criteria for MDD, Dysthymia, or Minor Depression. The completion rate for the 3-month follow-up was 94 percent. Because only a subgroup of the non-depressed patients was followed from only one study site, the health outcomes for this study cannot be considered randomized comparisons. Data were not presented on the baseline comparability between the follow-up sample and the original sample, or between the intervention and control groups among those in the follow-up sample, so we can not be as certain that follow-up group differences represent the intervention's effect.

According to the table of baseline characteristics, participants were primarily middle-aged females of Hispanic background and were largely low-income, with only 24 percent of the sample reporting annual incomes of $\geq$ $16,800 at that time (late 1990s). They also had high rates of positive screening tests (41 percent on the single-item screener and 33 percent on the CESD) and confirmed DSM-III-R depression diagnoses (13 percent).

This study found mixed results. Among patients who were depressed at baseline, patients in the two screening groups were more likely to have fully recovered from depression (i.e., reported $\leq$ one depression symptom) at 3-month follow-up than those who were not screened (48 vs. 27 percent, p<0.05). Among the entire follow-up sample, however, the proportion meeting DSM-III-R criteria for depression was similar in the combined screening groups (37 percent) and in the usual care group (46 percent) at three month follow-up (p=0.19), though they lacked adequate power to detect a population-level impact (n=218). Also, after controlling for baseline severity of depression (which differed between the screened and usual care groups in the full randomized sample), the mean reduction in DSM-III-R symptom counts was similar for the two groups (1.6 in screened vs. 1.5 in unscreened after controlling for baseline severity, p=0.21). While screening improved health outcomes in depressed patients, the effect was not large enough to create group differences at the level of the full follow-up sample. Since the follow-up sample included a considerably larger proportion of people who were depressed or symptomatic than the full sample, the effect would be even weaker in a full sample of primary care patients.

## Key Question 1a: What is the impact of clinician feedback of screening test results (with or without additional care management support) on depression response and remission in screen-detected depressed patients receiving primary care?

**Summary of findings.** Two good-quality[109,110] and six fair-quality[111-116] randomized controlled trials reported providing the impact of giving depression screening results to clinicians on health outcomes in screened populations (Table 5). Four of these studies involved general adult populations (N=1,908)[109,110,113,114] and four focused on older adults (N=1,443).[111,112,115,116] Four of these were also included in the previous review.[109-112] All studies randomized and/or enrolled patients who screened positive on at least one depression screening instrument which was often administered in the clinic waiting room. Although all patients were screened, feedback of screening test results was only given to providers of patients who screened positive (Appendix G Table 1).

In general adult populations, four trials screened a total of 38,843 primary care patients to detect 1,908 depressed adult patients (Table 5). Bergus and colleagues conducted a small, fair-quality RCT in a rural setting which did not support the effectiveness of screening programs with no depression care supports beyond simple feedback of screening results.[113] Another small, fair-quality RCT improved depressive symptomatology, but had a highly selected participant sample because they only enrolled screened adults with newly-detected depression (i.e., patients already known to be depressed were excluded from the trial, as were those who were actively seeking treatment for depression).[114] In this trial clinicians were given a detailed depression treatment protocol during the visit that included a recommended follow-up schedule and educational materials for the patient, and also received logistical support from other staff for scheduling follow-up visits and facilitating referrals. Two trials with considerably higher intensity interventions involving depression care by other staff were effective in improving depression outcomes,[109,110] particularly for adults with newly detected depression. These trials included such elements as intensive clinician and office support staff training, support staff or specialty mental health provider participation in ongoing depression care, and multiple follow-up contacts. See Table 6 for a summary of intervention elements included in each study. It was impossible to determine the degree to which the screening components contributed to the positive effects in the studies that also included additional depression care supports beyond simple screening and related interventions targeting the primary care provider.

In screening focused on older adults, four fairly large-scale trials screened 12,432 primary care patients to identify a total of 1,443 depressed older adults to test the impact of screening feedback with some care supports on remission and symptom reduction. The only trial with a significant treatment effect was also the only trial that expanded the role of other staff to provide depression management functions (in this case, assessment and regular follow-up). None of the trials in older adult patients limited enrollment to patients with newly identified depression. Intervention and usual care groups all showed some improvement from baseline, but only one of the four interventions in these trials improved depression remission rates or symptoms beyond usual care. The trial conducted in the Netherlands,[115] provided no extra care support beyond clinician training and provision of a treatment protocol consistent with Dutch depression care guidelines.[117] Although this trial did find an increase in the proportion of patients treated with antidepressants, no differences were found in depression remission or symptom severity at 12 months. Another trial offered a psychoeducational group to patients in addition to screening and provider feedback,[111] but patient participation in the psychoeducational group was minimal. The intervention group in this trial showed similar rates of depression remission and improvement to those who were simply screened without further intervention. The intervention in a third trial[112] included individually-tailored treatment recommendations, educational materials, and three scheduled follow-up visits with the provider. Adherence with follow-up visits was not reported. These supports were ineffective in a medically indigent, largely black, older adult population with multiple medical and psychiatric co-morbidities.[112]

Finally, the one trial[116] that did report an improvement in depression symptomatology among older patients who screened positive for depression involved the assistance of a case manager, who conducted an in-depth assessment and then referred the patient to primary or specialty care or to a multidisciplinary geriatric assessment team for further assessment. The case manager also provided patient education and follow-up. These results were reported in the subgroup of older adults screening positive for depression who were enrolled in a trial that attempted to identify patients with any of five high risk conditions. Therefore, this was not a randomized comparison, and the patient population was limited to patients who scored in a "high risk" range for a number of conditions. It was unclear if patients screening positive for depression only (i.e., none of the other four conditions screened for) could have been eligible for study inclusion. Thus, the generalizability of this trial to general primary care screening for depression in older adults may be limited.

**Study details.** All eight studies were conducted in outpatient primary care settings, seven in the United States and one in the Netherlands. Study settings included urban, rural, and indigent clinics, and two of the studies involved multiple geographic sites across of the US.[109,110] Four of the studies[111,112,115,116] focused on screening older adults and will be discussed separately from the others. In all studies, the usual care participants were screened as well as those in the intervention groups, often in the waiting room prior to a scheduled visit, but results of the screening tests were not systematically given to the providers of usual care patients or used in their care. The primary outcomes of two studies involved subgroup analyses,[109,116] which were therefore non-randomized (though controlled) comparisons. We included these analyses in our review because they were conducted in the context of a well-designed and implemented randomized controlled trials and were likely planned a priori.[109]

**Studies focusing on general adult patients.** Four studies focused on general adult populations. In a recent small (n=59) study in a rural setting,[113] providers at two private health clinics were educated about the PHQ-9. Researchers subsequently screened consecutive clinic patients. Patients with a positive score on the PHQ-9 were randomized either to have their PHQ-9 results given to their providers or not. Providers of intervention participants were asked to review the completed PHQ-9. No other depression care support was provided. Providers saw both intervention and control participants and therefore contamination is possible.

After 6 months there were no statistically significant group differences in either the proportion of participants in remission or in change in PHQ-9 score. This was a small study, however, with only 59 randomized participants. Even with their fairly good follow-up rate of 86 percent, there was minimal power to detect even large differences. For example, they found that 52 percent of the intervention group achieved remission from depression at 6-month follow-up, compared with 38 percent of the control group. The power for this comparison was approximately 10 percent, given their sample size. In order to achieve statistical significance with 80 percent power with their sample size, approximately 80 percent of the intervention participants would have to be in remission, compared with 38 percent of the control group. Thus, this study was not adequately powered to detect differences that would likely be clinically significant. They also reported differences in PHQ-9 score change, which is likely to have more power than the binomial comparison, but they did not report the standard deviations that would have allowed us to analyze the power for this analysis. This study also included a fairly large proportion of participants who were already taking medications for depression or anxiety (38 percent), though they do not specify the proportion taking antidepressants.

In another small (n=61) study with a largely indigent population,[114] Jarjoura and colleagues recruited patients from an internal medicine residency clinic who were either enrolled in Medicare or who were without private health insurance and had low income. Patients were excluded from this study if they were currently receiving treatment for any mental health problem (including depression), were seeking help for mental health problems, or reported suicidal ideation on the screening test. While there was a high background level of depression in the population, with positive screening test results for 45 percent of screened patients, only 9 percent of the screened patients were eligible for the study (i.e., had a positive screening test *and* were not already being treated for depression).

In the intervention condition, a screening nurse advised resident physicians of the positive screening results and provided a protocol outline asking the physician to: 1) explore symptoms with the patient and affirm screening results; 2) attempt to rule out physical conditions, medications, or other primary psychiatric diagnoses; 3) provide information, treatment, and follow-up at specified intervals; and 4) facilitate refer to behavioral treatment. Control participants who screened positive were informed they might have a problem with depression and that effective treatments were available. Participants were contacted at 6- and 12-months after the baseline visit and 90 percent completed at least one follow-up interview.

Researchers reported that intervention status predicted change in Beck Depression Inventory (BDI) in a mixed model linear regression. At six-month follow-up, average BDI score for the treatment group had improved by 7.6 points more than that of the control group (p<0.05, BDI range 0-63). Intervention effects were maintained at 12 months, with BDI score improvement in the intervention group 6.5 points greater than in the control group (p=0.03). As with the Bergus et al[113] study, this was a small study that randomized individuals rather than providers (and was therefore vulnerable to contamination). This study, however, used an analysis technique likely to have more power than the Bergus et al analyses.

This study limited the sample to those who were not being treated for depression at baseline, thus eliminating patients who were diagnosed with depression but were untreated, under-treated, or resistant to treatment. The intervention in the Jarjoura et al[114] study did provide elements beyond simple feedback to a provider, including a protocol and positive screening test results, but the program was not extremely extensive and involved a level of treatment that is feasible for many or most primary care settings. A total of 70 percent of the patients in the intervention condition were given depression care (24 percent received mental health specialty care, with or without antidepressants, and an additional 45 percent received antidepressants without specialty care), compared with only 15 percent in the usual care condition, none of whom received specialty mental health care. Thus, the combination of limiting the program to newly detected depression and moderate levels of support appeared to be sufficient to improve patients' depression.

Two large-scale studies[109,110] included extensive interventions beyond screening. Both included study sites in many regions of the US and both used a two-step screening approach adapted from the Composite International Diagnostic Interview (CIDI), where depressive symptoms are only explored if the patient is positive on a two-item initial screener. One of the studies[110] found significant group differences in depressive symptomatology and remission, while the other found a benefit only among the subgroup of newly detected patients with depression.[109]

The study by Wells[110] and colleagues randomized clinics to usual care or one of two extensive quality-improvement interventions for depression care. One intervention condition (QI-Meds, referred to as IG1 in Table 5) included screening; institutional monetary commitment; staff and clinician training (1- or 2-day workshops); clinician manuals; monthly training lectures; academic detailing; numerous materials for clinicians, staff, and patients; initial visit with nurse specialist for assessment, education, and discussion of patients preferences and goals; and trained nurse specialists for follow-up assessment and on-going support for medication adherence for those prescribed antidepressant medications. The other intervention condition (QI-Therapy, referred to as IG2 in Table 5) included all of the same QI elements as the QI-Meds condition except that it included trained therapists to provide manualized CBT and reduced co-pay for those referred for psychotherapy, rather than nurse specialists to support medication adherence. Providers in both intervention groups were expected to provide the treatment they deemed most appropriate for each patient, so patients in both groups could have received antidepressants or mental health specialty care. For example, referrals to mental health specialists ranged from 63 percent to 89 percent in the QI-therapy clinics and between 17 and 45 percent in the QI-Meds clinics. Structured follow-up sessions with a nurse medication specialist on the phone or in person averaged 1.8 sessions for patients in the QI-Therapy and 5.1 for QI-Meds patients.

Medical directors of the usual care clinics were mailed the AHRQ depression practice guidelines with quick reference guides for distribution to clinicians. Patients in control clinics were screened and patients were told that while they could inform their providers of the screening test results, the study staff would not send the results to their providers. Patients who screened positive on the CIDI were enrolled in the interventions and followed up.

At follow-up, the proportion of participants in either treatment arm who were still positive on the CIDI 2-item screener was 40 percent at 6 months and 42 percent at 12 months, while 50 percent of usual care participants still scored positive on the CIDI at 6 months and 51 percent at 12 months (p=0.001 for group differences at 6 months, p=0.005 at 12 months). At 5-year follow-up, program benefits were sustained for the QI-therapy group, which had positive CIDI screening scores of 36 percent of the intervention participants compared with 44 percent of the usual care participants (p=0.05). The difference between the control and QI-meds group was not significant at 5-year follow-up (38 vs. 44 percent positive, p=0.08).[118] These results provide good evidence for the effectiveness of their program. It is impossible to determine, however, what role, if any, the screening component played in the success of their program, which included so many elements. Further, while this intervention was proven feasible for primary care settings, it involved significant institutional commitment and may not reflect the care that would be found currently in most settings.

The Rost et al study[109] was designed for practices without ready access to mental health specialty care and also contained extensive care support elements beyond screening. Researchers cluster-randomized clinics to usual care or an intervention in which office staff recruited, screened, and enrolled participants who screened positive prior to a clinic visit. If the physician confirmed the depression diagnosis, the participant was scheduled for a return visit with the physician and to meet with the nurse specialist in one week. The nurse specialist reassessed the patient's level of depression, discussed treatment options and preferences, and asked the participant to complete a homework assignment. Participants completed up to eight additional sessions following the same pattern, either by phone or a face-to-face visit. Nurse documentation logs indicated that the nurses intervened in 92.5 percent of the patients in the intervention condition, contacting these patients an average of 5.2 times. Physicians and nurses in the intervention clinics were also trained in depression assessment and treatment and had access to free 24-hour consultation for patient-specific questions.

Although there was a significant overall treatment effect,[119] outcome data were only presented in two strata: patients who were not already being treated for depression ("newly identified"), and patients who were already or had recently been treated for depression ("recently treated"). Among the newly identified, CESD scores dropped an average of 21.7 points in the intervention group and only 13.5 points in the control group (p<0.05). In the recently treated, CESD scores dropped in both groups and did not differ between groups. At 2-year follow-up, significantly fewer of the newly identified patients in the intervention group met CESD screening criteria for depression (26 percent), compared with the control group (59 percent) (p<0.05). As with the Wells study, the effect of the screening component cannot be isolated.

**Studies focusing on older adult patients.** Four fair-quality, cluster-randomized RCTs focused on older adults.[111,112,115] A 2006 study conducted in the Netherlands randomized 34 general practices (GP) to intervention or usual care conditions.[115] Providers in the intervention practices attended a 4-hour training session on diagnosis and treatment of late-life depression, with a treatment protocol based on Dutch treatment guidelines.[117] In all practices, patients aged 55 or older were screened for depression with the Geriatric Depression Scale (GDS), and those scoring five or greater underwent a diagnostic evaluation using the Primary Care Evaluation of Mental Disorders (PRIME-MD). Usual care providers were not informed of screening test or PRIME-MD results. The intervention providers were informed of screening results and conducted the PRIME-MD interview themselves to determine MDD diagnosis. Patients with MDD diagnoses who were not currently using antidepressants were invited to participate in the study.

Fifteen percent of the 3,937 patients screened scored five or greater on the GDS, and 53 percent of the 339 consenting to the diagnostic interview were diagnosed with MDD and enrolled in the study. At 12-month follow-up, the groups did not differ on either proportion depressed or on symptom severity scores. Fifty-seven percent of the intervention group participants and 52 percent of the usual care participants still met criteria for depression at the 12-month follow-up.

Whooley and colleagues[111] randomized HMO primary care clinics to either an intervention or control condition. The intervention condition involved screening, feedback, treatment guidelines, and training for providers and group psycho-educational classes offered to patients and families. The control condition also involved screening and the clinics received the same one-hour training session. Patients were screened with the Geriatric Depression Scale (GDS) and 14 percent of the participants screened positive for depression and were enrolled in the study, with 20 percent receiving antidepressants during the previous year. Although this study included group classes, only 12 percent of the patients attended them. Follow-up after 2 years revealed improvements in both groups with no differences between the intervention and control groups.

Callahan and colleagues[112] randomized clinical practices to usual care or to a program screening for depression, dementia, and alcoholism. Providers in the intervention group received a letter for each of their study patients screening positive on two separate depression instruments. These letters contained the results of the second screening test, a list of medications that may cause depressive symptoms, and treatment recommendations. This letter was placed in the patient's chart, along with handouts for the patient. The provider was encouraged to schedule three appointments with the patient over the course of the next three months. Completion rates for visits were not reported. Providers in the control group were given no information or screening results, and additional appointments were left to the discretion of the provider. Providers in both groups were given an educational session on late-life depression and completed surveys after baseline visits of study patients. Sixteen percent of the patients in this study screened positive on the first screener, the Center of Epidemiologic Studies Depression Scale (CESD), and of these, 28.6 percent completed and were positive on the Hamilton Depression Rating Scale (HAMD). No group differences were found at 6 or 9 months follow-up, with very few patients in either group (12 to 13 percent) achieving remission. The patient population was an indigent, urban, largely Black group of seniors with co-morbid medical and psychiatric illnesses and significant functional disability at baseline.

Rubenstein and colleagues[116] conducted a non-randomized controlled trial in which patients in two VA clinical practices aged 65 or older were screened via a postal survey for five different common geriatric conditions (depression, falls/balance problems, urinary incontinence, memory loss, and functional impairment). Those scoring in the "high risk" range (indicating impairment on four or more of the ten items on the screening instrument) were invited to enroll in the trial. Participants at the clinical practice assigned to the control group received usual care, though if a serious condition was identified then the patient's primary care provider was notified. Participants in the clinical practice assigned to the intervention group were contacted by a case manager, who performed a more thorough assessment over the telephone. After completing the assessment, the case manager provided referrals to primary or specialty care providers, as needed, or for further evaluation by a multidisciplinary geriatric assessment team. The case manager also provided patient education, a written summary of recommendations, scheduled appointments, and conducted follow-up calls (one-month post-assessment and then quarterly). Overall, 42 percent of those returning questionnaires scored as "high-risk", 79 percent (n=792) of these enrolled in the study, and 41 percent of the enrolled scored in the depressed range on the GDS (45.8 percent of those completing the GDS).

Among the entire enrolled population, including those who were not depressed at baseline, no differences were seen in change in depressive symptomatology over time. Among the 206 participants who were above the cut-off for likely depression on the GDS at baseline and completed the 12-month assessment, those in the intervention group showed a greater decline in depression severity after one year.

GDS scores of participants in the intervention group dropped by an average of 3.7 points, compared with an average decline of 2.7 points among control participants (p=0.05). However, only 72.5 percent of the sample completed the GDS at one-year, so despite the high follow-up rate for the study overall, the follow-up rate for this instrument was considerably lower. Also, we do not know if the intervention and control participants in the subgroup of participants meeting depression criteria at baseline were similar to each other, nor do we know what the follow-up rate was among these baseline depressed.

All studies of older adults were well-designed, fairly large-scale studies with apparently similar rates of background depression in their populations. Two studies focused additional supports on the treating provider in the form of education, screening, and feedback, with other elements such as repeat visits with the provider (Callahan) or outside psycho-educational classes for patients.[111] One utilized case managers rather than focusing on improving the care provided by the primary care clinician.

## Key Question 2: What are the harms of screening for depressive disorders in adults and older adults?

We did not find any studies that included adverse events of screening.

## Key Question 3: Is antidepressant and/or psychotherapy treatment of older depressed adults effective in improving health outcomes?

**Summary of findings.** We found three good-quality systematic reviews in older adults[120-122]that each included meta-analyses (Table 7). One examined the efficacy of antidepressants,[121] one examined the efficacy of psychotherapy,[122] and one examined both types of treatments.[120] Two of these reviews[120,121] found that antidepressants were effective in treating depressed older adults, and approximately doubled the odds of remission compared with placebo controls, with OR of 2.03 (CI: 1.67, 2.46) for patients with major and minor depression; 2.13 (CI: 1.61, 2.86) for the community-dwelling subset; and 2.27 (CI: 1.72, 2.94) in the subset with MDD. Two good-quality meta-analyses[120,123]of psychotherapy effectiveness concluded that psychotherapy is effective in treating depression in older adults. Depressed older adults treated with psychotherapy were roughly two-and-a-half times more likely to achieve remission than those who were not treated with psychotherapy, with the ORs estimated at 2.47 (CI: 1.76, 3.47) and 2.63 (CI: 1.96, 3.53). Effect sizes estimates range from 0.72 to 1.09.

**Study details - antidepressants.** Numerous systematic reviews examining antidepressant efficacy in older adults have been published since the end of the previous USPSTF report's search window. We limited our inclusion to the two most recent good-quality systematic reviews that also included meta-analyses — a Cochrane review published in 2000[121] and another review published in 2006.[120] There was considerable overlap among the two included reviews, though they had somewhat different inclusion criteria and search windows and therefore different sets of included trials. Another good-quality review of newer antidepressant efficacy in adults was also published in 2000[75] and discussed efficacy in older adults separately. This study, however, overlapped substantially with the Cochrane review, and since the Cochrane review provided more detail, we excluded this other 2000 review.

The most recently published meta-analysis[120] examined 62 pharmacotherapy studies, 32 psychotherapy studies, and five studies examining both interventions in depressed older adults. This good-quality review included studies involving the full range of depressive disorders, including minor depression, dysthymia, and MDD. These authors included non-randomized comparative studies, although 89 percent of the included studies were randomized trials. All studies included a control condition and no restrictions were set with regard to setting (e.g., inpatient, outpatient, residential). In addition to providing overall results for all depressive disorders, they also reported the results of trials focusing exclusively on MDD separately. The authors combined all agents to determine overall effectiveness of antidepressants and combined all therapeutic modalities to determine overall effectiveness of psychotherapy. Of the 77 comparisons of clinician-reported outcomes, the specific agents examined included roughly the same number of reports for SSRIs (21/77) and TCAs (22/77), and over one third of the drugs were categorized as "other," many of which were non-SSRI second generation medications.

This review found an overall effect size of antidepressants of 0.69 (CI 0.57, 0.81, k=77 comparisons) for clinician-rated depression (most commonly the HAM-D) and 0.62 (CI 0.45, 0.79 k=28 comparisons) for self-rated depression. Although they do not report the absolute proportion of patients in the treatment and control groups whose depression remitted, the authors do report that treated participants were approximately twice as likely as control participants to go into remission (OR 2.03, CI: 1.67, 2.46). For studies focusing exclusively on MDD, clinician-rated depression had an effect size of 0.79 (CI: 0.64, 0.95, k=39 comparisons).

This review reported effect sizes separately for different classes of antidepressant agents, though they did not limit this analysis to studies focused on MDD. The authors report effect sizes ranging from 0.48 (SSRIs) to 0.93 (TCAs) for clinician-rated improvement, and report effect sizes ranging from 0.22 (SSRIs) to 0.83 (TCAs) for self-rated improvement.

The 2000 Cochrane Review[121] included randomized, placebo-controlled trials using antidepressants in the treatment of depression in older adults. The authors included studies of major and minor depression recruited from outpatient, community, institutional, and inpatient sources. They included 23 placebo-controlled, double-blind RCTs involving SSRIs, other second generation antidepressants, TCAs, and MAOIs, 17 of which were included in the meta-analysis. Eleven of the trials included in the meta-analysis were TCAs, and three of the trials involved second generation medications (fluoxetine and mirtazapine). Separate analyses were conducted for each of the medication categories, and separate analyses were conducted to determine the percent recovered at the end of the trial, continuous HAM-D scores, other observer rating scales, and discontinuation rates. For this review we limited our focus to recovery rates and HAM-D scores. Most of these studies measured treatment outcome at 3 to 8 weeks. This Cochrane review reported the number, proportion, and odds ratios of participants who were not recovered from depression at trial's end. We converted these numbers to report those who recovered from depression for ease of interpretation and comparison with other meta-analyses.

The most commonly reported outcome was the proportion of patients still depressed at the end of the study, which we converted to percent no longer depressed. Pooled fixed effects odds ratios were estimated for each medication type. A total of 365 patients treated with SSRIs were compared with 372 placebo controls in two trials with estimated OR of 1.96 (CI: 1.39, 2.78). One of these trials also reported differences in HAM-D change scores of 1.7 points in favor of the treatment group (CI:0.54, 2.60). Trials of other second generation antidepressants examined mirtazepine and two other medications not approved for use in the U.S. (minaprine, and medifoxamine), estimating an overall OR of 1.92 (CI: 1.07, 3.45) in 102 patients treated with active agents and 96 placebo controls in two trials. No HAM-D results were reported for either of these trials. For TCAs, 245 patients treated with TCAs were compared with 223 placebo controls in ten trials and had an estimated OR of 3.12 (CI: 2.13, 4.76). One trial reported that treatment participants improved on the HAM-D by 9.6 points (CI: 9.4, 13.8) more than the control participants. Analyses of MAOIs included a total of 58 patients treated with MAOIs and 63 with placebo in two trials, and found an OR of 5.88 (CI: 2.56, 14.28). No HAM-D results were reported for MAOIs. In terms of recovery rates, these studies found 28 to 49 percent of patients recovering from depression among antidepressant users and only 10 to 25 percent recovering in the placebo control groups.

In addition to overall results by medication type, they report meta-analysis results separately for outpatient/community recruitment, which are of greatest relevance to this review. Antidepressants were more effective than placebo, with 36 percent of antidepressant users recovered at the end of the study compared with 21 percent of the placebo patients, estimated OR of 2.13 (CI: 1.61, 2.86).

Although they did include some studies of hospitalized and institutionalized patients, most of these trials excluded a large proportion of those screened for inclusion due to comorbid physical illness or high levels of depression severity. Thus, the results of these analyses are best generalized to relatively healthy elders with mild- to moderate- depression severity, and only to very short-term outcomes.

**Study details - psychotherapy.** As with antidepressant therapy, several systematic reviews have been published examining psychotherapy efficacy in older adults since the end of the previous USPSTF report's search window. We limited our inclusion to the two most comprehensive recent good-quality systematic reviews of psychotherapy for depression in older adults, one by Pinquart and colleagues[120] and the other by Cuijpers and colleages[122], both published in 2006. While there was substantial overlap between the two reviews, their inclusion and exclusion criteria led to somewhat different bodies of evidence and we therefore included both reviews.

The Pinquart review did not report search dates, but appeared to have covered the literature through 2004. It included studies in which participants had a median age of 60 or greater, required a placebo or no-treatment control group, and included non-randomized comparisons, for a total of 32 trials. They report results separately for clinician-rated and self-report outcomes. The Cuijpers review searched an additional year (through 2005), included trials of participants aged 50 or greater, included trials that compared two active treatments as well as those that included control groups, and only included randomized comparisons, for a total of 25 trials. Pinquart and colleagues specifically reported including non-English language studies. No mention of language restriction was reported in the Cuijpers report, and no non-English language studies were among the list of included trials. Most of the 13 studies included in Pinquart but not in Cuijpers appeared to be non-randomized controlled trials and non-English language trials. Most of the 12 trials included in Cuijpers but not in Pinquart were either comparative effectiveness trials (i.e., they did not include a no-treatment control group) or were published after 2004.

The systematic review and meta-analysis by Pinquart and colleagues[120] found an overall effect size of 1.09 (CI: 0.91, 1.26, k=35 comparisons) for clinician-rated depression severity (usually using the HAM-D) and 0.83 (CI: 0.69, 0.98, k=52 comparisons) for self-rated depression. Twenty-six of the comparisons of clinician-rated depression involved some form of cognitive behavioral therapy. The other comparisons involved problem-solving, reminiscence, interpersonal, rapid eye movement, or life review therapy. Likewise, more then three-fourths of the comparisons involving self-reported outcomes used cognitive behavioral therapy. While they do not report the absolute proportion of patients in the treatment and control groups whose depression remitted, they do report that treated participants were more than twice as likely to go into remission (OR 2.47, CI: 1.76, 3.47). For studies focusing exclusively on MDD (excluding dysthymia and minor depression), clinician-rated depression had an effect size of 0.96 (CI: 0.69, 1.23, k=16 comparisons).

The review by Cuijpers and colleagues[122] reported an effects size of 0.72 (CI: 0.59, 0.85) for psychological treatment of depression in older adults, among trials that included a control condition (k=21 comparisons). This is within the 95 percent confidence interval of the Pinquart study for self-reported depression. This review did not report clinician- and self-reported symptomatology separately, but instead averaged these two measures if a trial reported both types of outcomes, and combined both types of outcomes in a single meta-analysis. Thus, this effect size reflects a blend of clinician report (which tends to show larger effects) and self-report (which tends to show smaller effects). Half of the comparisons in this review involved cognitive behavioral therapy, and the remaining involved behavior therapy alone, reminiscence or life-review, interpersonal, problem solving, or "other" therapies. Eleven studies in the Cuijpers review included remission rates, usually based on falling below a pre-specified cut-off on a continuous depression measure. They calculated an overall OR of 2.63 (CI: 1.96, 3.53), which is well within the 95 percent confidence interval for remission in the Pinquart review. Thus, these two reviews reported very consistent results for remission, but the average degree symptom improvement was somewhat smaller in the Cuijpers review than the Pinquart review, and this may in part be due to the method of analyzing the outcomes. It is also possible that randomized trials result in smaller group differences than non-randomized controlled trials, though the data were not presented that would allow us to verify this hypothesis.

## Key Question 4: What are the adverse effects of antidepressant treatment (particularly SSRIs and other second-generation drugs) for depression in adults and older adults?

**Summary of findings.** We examined serious adverse effects associated with antidepressant treatment including: suicide-related events (completed suicide, serious self-harm or attempted suicide, suicidal ideation) and serious psychiatric events, including hospitalization. Since adverse effects— typically nausea, dizziness, diarrhea, headache, sexual dysfunction, or insomnia— occur in 61 percent of patients during clinical trials of antidepressant medications,[57,92] we examined rates of early discontinuation, particularly discontinuations due to adverse effects. For older adults, we also considered evidence of serious medical events (e.g., upper gastrointestinal bleeding) associated with SSRIs and other second-generation antidepressant use.

*Suicide-related event rates* were most commonly reported per person receiving treatment, without consideration of exposure time. Event rates per 10,000 persons for three suicide-related outcomes are reported in Table 8: for *completed suicide*, for *suicidal behaviors* (usually defined to include suicide attempts, preparatory acts, or nonfatal, serious self-harm), and *for suicidal behaviors and ideation* combined. Table 9 reports risk differences in these outcomes for patients with MDD.

For *completed suicide,* none of the seven meta-analyses of short-term trials in adults being treated either for MDD or for any psychiatric indications supplied clear evidence that use of second-generation antidepressants— or of SSRIs in particular— significantly increased rates of completed suicide for those on antidepressant treatment compared with placebo. However, despite the large sample sizes, there were very few suicides (7 to 43 total suicides among treated and control patients per review) which limited power to detect these rare events; using reported or calculated OR, these results are compatible with no increase in short-term risk, some protective effect, or some increased risk. Most meta-analyses estimated suicide rates ranging from 3.8 to 8.8 per 10,000 antidepressant-treated adults, compared with 2.3 to 9.3 per 10,000 placebo-treated patients. Two studies' data represented outliers. One FDA report estimated 1.8 completed suicides per 10,000 antidepressant-treated MDD patients (compared with 0.67 per 10,000 placebo-treated MDD patients);[124,125] this estimate is markedly lower than other studies and may reflect methodological differences (e.g., in how suicides and related events were categorized, among other differences). And, the much higher estimates of suicide rates in both antidepressant and placebo-treated patients in another review[126] could reflect the suicide risk among more severely depressed patients (since the majority of studies in this review employed active controls rather than placebos) as well as quality concerns with this review.

Three fair or good quality large observational studies reported on suicide with antidepressant treatment in a total of 383,796 patients from a large US HMO and from GP practices in the UK.[127-129] Among the two highest quality studies reporting a 6-8 month follow-up duration, crude suicide rates were 4.7 and 4.8 per 10,000 persons treated primarily with second-generation antidepressants, with slightly higher rates reported among children and adults under 30 years. These studies also indicate higher risk for suicide death among men compared with women. Although these observational studies do not give us comparative information for people who were not taking antidepressants, they give credence to the estimate of approximately 4/10,000 suicide cases among antidepressant users found most consistently in the meta-analyses of short-term trial data.

For ***suicidal behaviors*** (defined differently across studies, but usually including suicide attempts, preparatory acts, or serious self-harm), results from five meta-analyses did not show significant differences in the odds of suicidal behaviors in adults treated with antidepressants compared with placebo, with several exceptions. One fair quality systematic review indicated an increased odds of suicidal behaviors in adults of all ages being treated with SSRIs for any indication (OR 2.70; CI: 1.22, 6.97);[130] this report was limited to published studies only and did not have clear adverse event ascertainment for the majority of patients. In an FDA review of regulatory data of placebo-controlled trials, odds of suicidal behavior were approximately doubled in adults under age 25 taking second-generation antidepressants for all psychiatric disorders (OR 2.31; CI: 1.02, 5.64);[125] in contrast, the odds of suicidal behaviors was not changed among middle-aged adults, and was greatly reduced in older adults on second-generation antidepressants (OR 0.06, CI: 0.01, 0.58).[124]

The highest odds of non-fatal suicidal behavior was reported in adults of all ages being treated for MDD with paroxetine compared to placebo (OR 6.70; CI: 1.1, 149.4), with most events (8/11) occurring in those aged 18-29 years.[131] The NNT-harm for this estimate is 373 (CI: 208, 1818).

Two good quality observational studies suggest that, in contrast to a higher risk of suicide deaths in men, there were no sex differences in risks of self-harm, but there were age-related differences.[128,129] Suicide attempts were significantly greater in younger persons (under aged 18 years),[129] with a higher rate of self-harm in those aged 19-30.[128] The highest risk for suicidal behaviors occurred in the month prior to treatment initiation and the first month of treatment.[129] Rate of suicidal behaviors in real-world practice situations was similar to trial rates for one study[129] but was substantially higher in the other;[128] this higher rate could reflect real differences or perhaps represents study differences in definitions (and perhaps ascertainment).

For ***suicidal ideation***, three meta-analyses used a combined endpoint (suicidal ideation or behavior) and found no differences between antidepressant and placebo-treated patients, except for a reduction in older adults treated with second-generation antidepressants for all psychiatric conditions (OR 0.39;CI: 0.18, 0.78).[125]

For ***serious psychiatric events***, we did not find any existing systematic reviews and found very limited reliable primary evidence to estimate mania precipitation or to distinguish other uncommon but important psychiatric side-effects from suicide-related behaviors.

For ***tolerability***, we found eight systematic reviews that reported overall discontinuation rates and discontinuation due to adverse effects as measures of the impact of adverse effects associated with antidepressants,[72,75,90-95] and two large cohort or uncontrolled treatment trials.[46,96] Early treatment discontinuation ranged from 16 to 29 percent in meta-analyses of antidepressant trials in primary care patients with depression, with a best estimate of 20 to 23 percent in "real-world" trials of primary care. Early discontinuations due to adverse effects were lower (5 to 12 percent). Patients aged 55 and older had higher discontinuation rates overall (27 to 36 percent) and for adverse effects (17 to 22 percent). With longer follow-up, adverse event discontinuation rates increased, particularly in those who switched or augmented medications due to lack of efficacy or intolerable side-effects.

As reported above, ***older adults*** were at lower risk for suicide-related harms during antidepressant treatment. For those over 65 years, antidepressant treatment was protective for both suicidal behaviors (OR 0.06; CI: 0.01, 0.58) and combined suicidal behaviors and ideation (OR 0.37; CI: 0.18, 0.76). For serious medical events in older adults, we found a fair-quality systematic review of six large observational studies from Denmark, Canada, the UK, and Holland examining bleeding risk in these SSRI's.[132] Among 26,005 Danish patients aged 16 years and older (almost half aged 60 or more years) risk for hospitalization for upper gastrointestinal (UGI) bleeding was increased compared with non-users during periods of current SSRI use only, with an excess risk of 3.1 per 1000 treatment years. In 317,824 Canadian patients 65 years and older on antidepressants, risk of hospitalization for UGI bleeding increased greatly with age, from 4.1 hospitalizations per 1000 person-years of SSRI treatment in those aged 65 to 70 years to 12.3 hospitalizations per 1000 person-years in octogenarians. Excess hospitalizations for UGI bleeding were increased five-fold (33.2 per 1,000 treatment years) in persons with prior UGI bleeding. In some, [133-135] but not all,[136] studies, odds of UGI bleeding among SSRI users were further increased at least two-to-three fold when SSRI users were also taking NSAIDs, with a lesser risk associated with co-use of aspirin or other anticoagulant medications.

**Study details.**

*Suicide and related-events, systematic reviews and meta-analyses of short-term trials*

For suicide-related events, we included two recent related reviews reported by the U.S. Food and Drug Administration (FDA),[124,125] an earlier FDA review,[137] and two reviews sponsored or in response to the Medicines and Healthcare Products Regulatory Agency (MHRA) in the United Kingdom,[105,131] along with a related review [138] and a related letter to the editor providing additional data.[139] Two additional reviews evaluated clinical trials submitted to regulatory agencies for drug approval by the U.S. FDA[126] or by the Medicines Evaluation Board of Netherlands.[140] One systematic review evaluated published clinical trials only.[130] We included all regulatory agency or related reviews, as well as systematic reviews, reporting on suicide-related events with antidepressant usage, unless the review was clearly updated by a more current review. These ten publications group together into seven main sets of data as shown in Table 8.

These reviews were generally large, reviewing 57 to 702 RCTs (with an average of 326 RCTs) and summarizing the experience of 5433 to 99,839 patients (41,379 patients on average). Most trials were less than 6 to 8 weeks and trial dropout rates were rarely considered but, where reported, exceeded 25 percent drop-out in about half of the trials. The limited reporting of methods to ensure systematic study retrieval and minimal information about individual study details in regulatory and related reviews, made it unclear where there was duplication. Lack of detailed reporting of methods and lack of criteria for quality rating regulatory (as opposed to systematic) reviews also impaired our effort to quality rate these reviews. Thus we provide no quality rating of regulatory and related reviews, but comment on possible concerns related to review methods and reporting. All reviews examined RCTs comparing SSRIs and other second-generation antidepressants with placebo (some trials also with active controls), but varied in whether they included both published and unpublished studies. We found it important to consider reviews including both published and unpublished trials to address potential bias found in previous reviews of only published trials of antidepressants.[141] Inclusion of unpublished data also helps minimize a potential non-reporting bias associated with trial sponsorship by the manufacturer.[142] We supplemented harms information available from meta-analyses of short-term efficacy trials conducted for drug approval with seven large observational studies.[127-129,143-146] These studies reported on risks in those with antidepressant use with a minimum of six months of follow-up conducted in the United States, UK or Denmark. Some of these also provided information on suicide rates in patients who were not taking antidepressant medications. Three studies which were rated fair or good quality are summarized in the text and Table 8,[127-129] with details on the fair to poor studies in Appendix G Table 8.[144-147]

**2006 FDA Report:**[124,125] This report conducted for the FDA provided the most current data and compared the risk of either suicidal behavior (e.g., suicide, suicide attempts, or preparatory acts) or suicidality (ideation or suicidal behavior) in a series of meta-analyses of 372 randomized placebo-controlled trials of 11 second-generation antidepressants (buproprion, citalopram, duloxetine, escitalopram, fluvoxamine, fluoxetine, nefazodone, paroxetine, sertraline, mirtazapine, and venlafaxine). Meta-analyses were based on individual and on trial-level data. Most adult patients (63 percent) were enrolled in SSRI trials. Sponsors (manufacturers) created datasets from all relevant trials by protocol and coded adverse events hierarchically with the most specific and serious suicide-related event that occurred for each subject superseding all others (e.g., completed suicide superseded suicide attempt which superseded preparatory acts which superseded ideation). However, in some cases this meant that suicidal ideation superseded self-injurious behaviors (intent unknown) and fatal or non-fatal events with insufficient information. Data were not provided to determine in how many cases suicidal ideation (a cognitive act) was coded instead of actual injurious behaviors or fatal or non-fatal events. Sponsors classified all events and prepared, but were not required to submit, narrative summaries for all "possibly suicide-related events." Events were limited to those occurring during the double-blind phase of treatment or within one day of stopping randomized treatment.

The FDA review included 99,839 adult patients being treated for major depressive disorder (MDD) and other psychiatric and behavioral disorders, with 15,505 person-years of observation for all participants. MDD was the most common indication (46 percent), followed by other psychiatric disorders (28 percent), other behavioral disorders (14 percent), other indications (9 percent), and non-MDD depression (4 percent). There were a total of eight suicides, 134 attempted suicides, 10 individuals with preparatory actions but no attempts, and 378 individuals with ideation only. Numbers of patients and event-rates were not reported for the other types of fatal and non-fatal possibly suicide-related events that were superseded by suicidal ideation.

Rates of suicide and suicide-related events were relatively more common in those with MDD. Patients with MDD (n= 37,252) accounted for most of the suicides (five of eight suicides), resulting in higher crude suicide rates (1.79 per 10,000 MDD patients treated with any of the 11 antidepressants over an average of 7.5 weeks) compared with patients being treated for other psychiatric disorders (0.66 suicides per 10,000 persons treated) or MDD patients on placebo (0.67 per 10,000 treated).[124] Similarly, other suicide-related events (suicidal attempts, preparatory behaviors, or ideation) were relatively more common in those with MDD than other psychiatric disorders (Appendix G Table 3). Thus, event rates and risk differences are reduced in analyses that combine the two groups (MDD with other psychiatric disorders in the category "all psychiatric indications"), but relative measures should not be distorted since the relative impact on all suicide-related events across treatment groups were similar in the two groups of patients.

Of greater importance, the primary outcome used in most meta-analyses, which was likely selected to improve power, was a combined outcome of the impact of medication on ideation and the impact on behaviors (suicidality, reflecting suicidal behaviors OR ideation). However, the direction of the impact of treatment compared with placebo was in opposite directions depending on whether the outcome was suicidal behaviors or suicidal ideation (Appendix G Table 3). For suicide-related behaviors, event rates tended to either be similar in those on active drug and placebo or to be reduced in the placebo groups. In contrast, for suicidal ideation, event rates tended to be higher in placebo than in the drug treatment groups. Because suicidal ideation occurred much more frequently than suicidal behavior, however, the results for the primary outcome are primarily influenced by the medications' impact on suicidal ideation rather than behaviors. Thus, this combined primary outcome can neither clearly differentiate the impact of antidepressant medications on ideation vs. behaviors, nor provide a clear a picture about the more critical impact of antidepressant medications on suicidal behaviors.

Therefore, to the extent possible, we focus on analyses from this report that reported on the outcome of suicidal behaviors (suicides, attempts, or preparation) in MDD (the highest risk group and most appropriate for absolute rates relevant to this report) and on patients with all psychiatric indications (higher power for relative measures of effect) (Tables 8 and 9).

Compared with placebo, patients with MDD taking active drug had no difference in the odds of suicide (OR 2.66, CI: 0.26, 130.9) or in the odds of suicidality (including ideation and behaviors) (OR 0.86; CI 0.67, 1.10) Similarly, there were no differences in completed suicides, suicidal behaviors or suicidality in active treatment vs. placebo among those with psychiatric indications. There were no differences in suicidal behaviors between drug classes (e.g., SSRIs, SNRIs, other modern antidepressants) in adults with psychiatric indications. However, there was heterogeneity of treatment risk within SSRIs: compared with placebo, suicidal behavior was more likely for those treated with paroxetine (OR 2.76; CI:1.16, 6.6) and less likely for those treated with sertraline (OR 0.25; CI: 0.07, 0.90) Cautions are advised in interpreting these numbers, due to multiple comparisons and since comparisons between medications are indirect comparisons which may also reflect differences across trials.[124] When examined by age, adults with psychiatric disorders under age 25 who were treated with second-generation antidepressants had the highest rates of suicidal behavior (60.4 per 10,000 persons) and significantly increased odds of suicidal behavior (OR 2.31; CI:1.02, 5.64), but not suicidality (ideation or behavior) (OR 1.55; CI: 0.91, 2.70), compared with those randomized to placebo. In adults aged 25-64, suicidality (ideation or behavior) was significantly reduced in those on second-generation antidepressants (OR 0.79; CI: 0.64, 0.98), but there was no impact on suicidal behavior alone (OR 1.03; CI: 0.68, 1.58). In contrast, older adults (ages 65 years or older) on these medications had a reduction in both suicidal behavior (OR 0.06; CI: 0.01, 0.58) and broader suicidality (OR 0.39; CI 0.18, 0.78). For all types of suicide-related events (suicide, attempts, preparatory acts, and ideation), differences between treatment groups were greatest in the 18-24 years and the 65 years and older age groups. In the older age group, rates for all events were lower in the antidepressant treated group than in placebo.

**Hammad 2006:**[137] In another FDA regulatory analysis of earlier data, the risk of completed suicide during short-term (6-17 week) treatment was examined using 2 placebo-controlled trials conducted as part of the drug development programs for five SSRIs (citalopram, fluoxetine, fluvoxamine, paroxetine, sertraline) and four other second-generation antidepressants (buproprion, mirtazapine, nefazodone, venlafaxine). Events were ascertained during active treatment only. Among adults with MDD (n=40,028 in 207 trials) or with anxiety disorders (n=10,972 in 44 trials), there were 21 and two completed suicides, respectively, with a mean exposure time of 1.4 patient-months. Rates of suicide in adults with MDD taking any second-generation antidepressant were 5.9 per 10,000 persons and 4.1 per 10,000 persons for those taking SSRIS, which did not differ significantly from suicide rates in placebo-treated patients with MDD. It is not clear why suicide rates were two to three times higher for both antidepressant- and placebo-treated patients with MDD in this review using drug development trial data, compared with the 2006 FDA report based on similar data. Several differences between the two reports are: 1) the time frame for data; 2) the inclusion of active controlled trials without a placebo arm in this review, but not 2006 FDA report (and the higher suicide rates in active control trials, perhaps due to patient severity); 3) a difference in included medications (duloxetine and escitalopram were not included in this report). In general, however, suicide rates in this report are consistent with the other systematic reviews and regulatory reviews.

**Khan 2003:**[126] This review of regulatory data obtained summary reports used as the basis of FDA approval for five SSRIs (citalopram, fluvoxamine, fluoxetine, paroxetine, and sertraline) to determine suicide risk in SSRI users; these reports summarized an unreported number of clinical trials submitted for regulatory approval from January 1985 to January 2000. Information on trial setting or included patients is lacking except that patients did not have psychotic features and had never had hypomania or mania. Suicides were assigned to the drug the person was taking at the time of the event, even if the trial primarily addressed another medication. It was not clear how those who discontinued treatment were classified. Suicide rates were 14.6 per 10,000 persons among SSRI users and 10.2 per 10,000 users among placebo, which were not significantly different. These suicide rates are much higher than those reported in other reviews, particularly considering that patients with all indications may have been included. However, the relative predominance of active controls, compared with placebo controls, among these trials suggests that these were more severely ill patients (as more severely ill patients would be less likely to be enrolled in trials with placebo treatment).

**MHRA Regulatory** [105,131] **and Other Related Reviews:** [138,139] The Medicines and Healthcare products Regulatory Agency (MHRA) and the Committee on the Safety of Medicine in the United Kingdom requested analytic work on suicides, non-fatal self-harm, and suicidal thoughts with use of SSRIs which has been reported in peer-reviewed publications[138,139] and technical reports.[105,131] This work examines 439 placebo-controlled trials submitted for regulatory approval providing data on six SSRIs (citalopram, escitalopram, fluoxetine, fluvoxamine, paroxetine, sertraline) in a total of 52,503 patients treated for all indications for a mean of 8-10 weeks (with patient numbers varying by analysis). A total of sixteen suicides, 203 episodes of non-fatal self-harm, and 177 reports of suicidal thoughts occurred.

Results among all adults suggested no impact of SSRI treatment on completed suicides (OR 0.85; 95 percent credible interval 0.20, 3.40), on non-fatal self-harm (OR 1.21; CI: 0.87, 1.83), or on suicidal thoughts (OR 0.80; CI: 0.49, 1.30). Due to data limitations, this study included suicides from fluoxetine trials in the self-harm category rather than the suicide category. The suicide rate in patients taking SSRIs (except fluoxetine) was 3.8/10,000 persons, compared with 4.1/10,000 persons in those on placebo. Although not significantly different, the direction of the main effect of treatment compared with placebo in suicide-related behaviors (increased), was opposite the main effect in suicidal ideation (decreased), which is consistent with the FDA reports described above. Meta-analyses were not conducted at the patient level and thus weren't stratified by trial type or adjusted for issues such as disease severity, age, or suicidal history. The proportion of patients with MDD vs. other indications could not be determined. This study did not include studies other than those submitted to the MHRA by the manufacturers, which could exclude trials conducted for non-regulatory reasons with less favorable adverse effects findings. However, given the large sample sizes needed for these rare outcomes, it is unlikely that there are independent investigators conducting large trials considering suicide or related events, and none were located during our systematic searches.

Looking specifically at paroxetine, data from 57 placebo-controlled RCTs of paroxetine treatment in 5433 adults with MDD were made available by the manufacturer.[131] Definitive suicidal behavior (without any fatalities) was increased in those on paroxetine relative to placebo (OR 6.7; CI: 1.1, 149.4), and eight of 11 events of suicidal behavior occurred in young adults (18-29 years). The risk difference for suicidal behavior was 26.8 per 10,000 (CI: 5.5, 48.0), with a NNT-H of 373 (CI: 208, 1818). When suicidal behavior and ideation were considered together, there was no significant difference between those on paroxetine and those on placebo (OR 1.3; CI: 0.7, 2.80).

**Fergusson:** [130] This fair quality systematic review of 411 published, randomized, placebo-controlled trials of five SSRIs (citalopram, fluoxetine, fluvoxamine, paroxetine, sertraline) in 18,413 adults treated for all indications for a mean of 10.8 weeks complements the MHRA review of regulatory data from the same time period (1967 through 2003). This review included the same SSRIs as the MHRA review, except for escitalopram, which was only included in the MHRA review. The number of patients and events were much smaller in this review of short-term trials that were published only: a total of seven suicides and 29 attempts in 18,413 patients. Rates of suicides (3.8 per 10,000 persons) were almost identical in this review and the MHRA review, but lack of similarity between the categorization of other suicide-related events prevents comparisons between these two meta-analyses. Rates of suicide did not differ between those on SSRI treatment and placebo (OR 0.95; CI: 0.24, 3.78). Combined fatal and non-fatal suicide attempts were increased in those on SSRIs, compared with placebo, (OR 2.28; CI: 1.14, 4.55), driven by the difference in non-fatal attempts (OR 2.70; CI: 1.22, 6.97). Adverse events may have been underreported given the reliance on published data only and since adverse event reporting was not available from the majority of trials. Also, almost half (46 percent) of trials had dropout rates of over 25 percent, which means adverse events were likely to have been missed, especially given that longer duration trials (7 weeks or longer) had an increased risk of fatal and non-fatal events. Even though this review included published trials only and half of patients in this review were in trials funded by the pharmaceutical industry, industry-funded trials reported an increased risk of fatal and non-fatal events with treatment compared with placebo while those funded by other sources did not.

**Storosum 2001:**[140] This review considered 85 short-term and longer-term clinical trials submitted to the Medicines Evaluation Board of the Netherlands from 1983-1997 for approval for use in major depression and another 14 placebo-controlled trials of antidepressant medications in those with MDD published from 1990-1999. Antidepressant drugs were not specified, but could have included nine second-generation antidepressants (bupropion, citalopram, fluoxetine, fluvoxamine, mirtazapine, nefazodone, paroxetine, sertraline, venlafaxine), if the Netherlands approval dates coincide with those in the US.[125] Rates of suicide in 77 short-term studies of patients with MDD were 8.8 per 10,000 persons treated with active drug, compared with 9.3 per 10,000 persons treated with placebo. Similarly, suicide attempts were not increased in those taking active drug compared with placebo. For all of these meta-analyses, the results are compromised by the type of trials available for review. The majority of trials were short-term efficacy designs that tend to screen out higher risk patients, including those at risk for suicide. None of these trials were designed to measure adverse effects, which is especially problematic for rare events such as suicide and events that may not be spontaneously reported such as suicide-related behaviors and ideation. As such, these analyses are plagued by issues related to power and measurement bias, particularly given the large dropout rates after which adverse events may not have been captured. Differences in event definition for analyses across meta-analyses complicates comparisons. Generalizability of this evidence is questionable due to very short time periods and that fact that participants differ from those seen in clinical practice in important ways: volunteers for studies generally have more mild to moderate depression; exclusion of those that are suicidal or at high risk upon entry to trial; and exclusion of those with comorbid psychiatric or medical illnesses. Therefore, we sought large observational studies and uncontrolled treatment studies in community settings as supplements.

### Suicide and related-events, cohort studies

We found seven large observational studies[128,129,143-146,148] from five separate practice or prescription data sources which reported adverse suicide-related events in a total of 1,064,603 patients receiving antidepressant prescriptions over 6 months to 5 years, plus 59,432 depressed patients who did not receive antidepressants. And, although many observational studies focused on comparative effectiveness, we were interested in absolute adverse event rates to determine the applicability of adverse event rates from the short-term clinical trials to primary care practice. Observational studies that could not supply absolute adverse event rates were not included. In observational pharmacoepidemiological studies, confounding by indication (e.g., the tendency of clinicians to prescribe drugs differentially based on disease severity, to give drugs that are less toxic in overdose, such as SSRIs, to their suicidal or more severe patients, or the tendency for clinicians to try newly available medications in treatment-resistant cases) is a major threat to validity for non-randomized drug-drug comparisons.[149] Data from several recent studies on antidepressant use in the community demonstrate that adjustment for potential confounders is not sufficient to remove all residual confounding by indication.[150,151] Given these quality concerns, we focus on the results from the three fair or good quality reports here,[127-129] with the remainder covered in Appendix G Table 8.[144-147]

**Simon 2006:**[129] In a good-quality cohort study in a large, prepaid, group practice from 1992-2003, suicides and attempts requiring hospitalization were assessed in 65,103 patients aged five to 105 years with diagnosed MDD, dysthymia, or depression NOS after their first dispense (for at least the prior 6 months) of any antidepressant. Patients could contribute more than one episode of "new" treatment. In the entire covered population, the suicide rate was 1.7 per 10,000 persons during this time period. There were 31 suicides and 76 suicide attempts requiring hospitalization during the 6 months after beginning "new" antidepressant treatments or 4.8 suicides per 10,000 persons treated and 11.7 suicide attempts per 10,000 treated. Men had higher odds of suicide death than women (OR 6.6; CI: 2.9, 14.7), with no variation across age nor across time from beginning treatment. Suicide attempts were greatly increased in those under age 18 (3.14 per 10,000 CI: 16, 46.8;) compared to those 18 years and over (7.8 per 10,000 persons, CI: 5.8, 9.8). There were almost as many serious suicide attempts during the six months preceding a "new" antidepressant as in the succeeding six months (76 and 73, respectively). Rates of suicide attempts remained the highest during the month preceding "new" treatment for adults and adolescents after excluding those with prior antidepressant treatments or suicidal attempts. Rates of suicide attempts were also increased in the month after starting "new" treatment compared with the subsequent five months (OR 2.4; CI: 1.6, 3.8), during which suicide attempts declined.

**UK General Practice Research Database**: Two studies utilized primary care records from the UK General Practice Research Database to examine harms associated with first dispense (for at least the prior 12 months) of antidepressants.[127,128] The more recent report using records from 1995-2001, which more fully represents the time period of use for second-generation antidepressants, was a good-quality cohort study evaluating suicides and self-harm events among 146,905 youth and adults aged 10 to 90 years (18 percent over 60 years) with diagnosed depression, dysthymia, or bipolar disorder after their first dispense of any of 26 first and second-generation antidepressants.[128] The median duration of follow-up was 0.66 years with an interquartile range of 0.57 to 1.03 and a total of 62,224 person-years for the whole cohort. In that time, 69 suicides occurred (56 in men and 13 in women; 19 in those aged 19 to 30 years) and 1,968 self-harm events. The self-harm events were primarily drug overdoses (81 percent). Thirty-six of the 69 patients who committed suicide (52 percent) were taking antidepressants at the time of their death. Outcomes were ascertained using death certificates along with diagnoses and reviewing free text notes from medical records. In those taking any antidepressant, the rate of suicide was 4.7 per 10,000 persons of all ages and 5.5 per 10,000 persons aged 19-30. The rate of self-harm was 134.7 per 10,000 persons of all ages and 214.7 in those aged 19-30 years. The standardized incidence rate for suicide (standardized to the age and sex of the UK population) was 6.2 (CI: 4.0, 8.5) per 10,000 person years, which was significantly higher in men (11.7 per 10,000 person-years) than women (0.9 per 10,000 person-years). In contrast, there was no sex difference in the standardized incidence rate for self-harm. Compared with those not exposed to antidepressants, unadjusted odds of suicide were increased three-fold or more in those with a history of self-harm, with referral to a mental health professional (possibly a proxy for more severe disease), with antipsychotic use, and with use of more than one antidepressant. Similarly, unadjusted odds of self-harm were increased three-fold or more in those with history of self-harm, with a mental health referral, with a comorbid alcohol misuse, and with use of more than one antidepressant. A fair-quality older study using similar methods and primary care records from 1988-1993, researchers examined suicide events for six months after dispenses of nine antidepressants (all first generation except for fluoxetine) for all indications.[127] There were 143 suicides among 172,598 persons taking antidepressants during 167,819 person-years of observation; the overall suicide rate was 8.5 (95 percent CI, 7.2, 10.0) per 10,000 person-years. Of the 143 individuals who committed suicide, 67 had a history of attempts (47 percent) and most (78 percent) had documented depressive illness.

***Serious psychiatric effects (hospitalization, mania precipitation).*** Very few studies were found. In a large good quality open-label effectiveness study of 2,876 screen detected outpatients with previously established non-psychotic major depressive disorder (in 18 primary care and 23 psychiatric community settings) treated with an SSRI (citalopram) under a protocolized treatment approach, 2 percent of patients experienced a serious psychiatric event (defined as suicidal ideation or hospitalization for worsening depression, substance abuse, suicidality, and other).[53] These data did not distinguish suicide-related harms from other serious psychiatric events. In another large fair-to-poor quality post-marketing study of primary care patients treated with one of six second-generation antidepressants, after exclusion of those with pre-existing mania, there were 1.2 reports of mania per 1000 patient-months of treatment within the first three months of treatment with no indication of the severity of the mania.[147]

***Tolerability.*** Although measurement methods are not very robust, a recent systematic review of comparative effectiveness of second-generation antidepressants reported that, on average, 61 percent of patients in efficacy trials of SSRIs and other second-generation antidepressants experience at least one adverse effect (e.g., nausea, headache, diarrhea, fatigue, dizziness, sexual dysfunction, tremor, dry mouth, or weight gain).[92] In a large fair to poor quality prescription event monitoring study of primary care patients,[147] nausea and vomiting, malaise, headache, dizziness, and drowsiness were reported in at least one-quarter of patients on one of six second-generation antidepressants during the first month of treatment. Since adverse event profiles appear to vary somewhat among medications that are equivalent in efficacy, clinicians may aim to minimize potential side-effects when choosing among first-line antidepressants.[92,129]

Early medication discontinuation is common, particularly in antidepressants, and can compromise expected benefits from treatment initiation. Since early discontinuation can result from several factors (e.g., lack of efficacy, intolerable side-effects, due to achieving complete treatment response), discontinuation due to adverse effects is a more accurate proxy for tolerability. Studies examining discontinuation due to adverse effects are detailed in Appendix G Table 6.

We located three at least fair quality systematic reviews or meta-analyses (in four publications) of mostly short-term (6-8 week) randomized controlled trials that compared SSRIs and/or other second generation antidepressant with placebo that reported overall discontinuation rates and discontinuation due to adverse effects for antidepressants and for placebo.[72,75,91,95] We included four additional, at least fair quality, comparative effectiveness reviews of short-term, head-to-head trials that reported on total and adverse effect-related discontinuation rates for second generation antidepressants.[90,92-94] Two fair-quality uncontrolled treatment trials[46,96] provided longer term (up to 10 months) discontinuation data. Five of the nine studies provided antidepressant discontinuation rates in primary care patients,[72,75,93,95,96] with one of these clearly conducted in community-based primary care.[96] Two reported data for older and younger patients separately.[90,94]

In trials of primary care patients with depression, short-term early discontinuation (within the first 2-3 months) for SSRIs for any reason ranged from 16 to 29 percent.[75,93,96] Short-term SSRI discontinuations from non-primary care populations fell within this range,[46,90-92] except for potentially higher total discontinuation rates in patients on higher doses (38 percent)[91] and in patients aged 55 years and older (27 to 36 percent).[90,94] These are unadjusted rates and most are based on relatively small numbers of patients, so any apparent age- or dose-related differences may not be statistically significant. Considering the data we found from "real-world" trials in primary care as best evidence, a reasonable best-case estimate of short-term overall SSRI discontinuation rate in primary care adults is 20 to 23 percent. As expected, with longer follow-up, total discontinuation for SSRIs increased to around 33 percent after 6 months.[96] Discontinuation after this time, however, could be due to remission (which is common after about 20 weeks) in both new and recurrent[152] patients, particularly in older studies in which treatment continuation beyond remission was not emphasized to clinicians.[57]

Discontinuation due to adverse events in primary care patients taking SSRIs and other second generation antidepressants ranged from 5 to 12 percent during the first 3 months.[72,93,95] Short-term antidepressant discontinuations from non-primary care populations fell with in the same range[90-92] or were higher in some studies of specific SSRIs or doses (14 to 16 percent)[46,91] and in patients aged 55 years and older (17 to 22 percent).[90,94] People who switched or augmented medications after lack of efficacy or intolerable side-effects in initial treatment had increased rates of discontinuation through each successive treatment regimen (up to 30 percent in 8 to 10 weeks), possibly indicating more severe or treatment resistant disease.[46] In community-based primary care, 26 percent of SSRI users discontinued use at 9 months due to adverse events.[96] These are unadjusted rates and most are based on relatively small numbers of patients, so any apparent differences may not be statistically significant.

### Older adults.

**Adverse events:** We found no admissible evidence focused solely on older adults for suicidality, serious psychiatric effects, and discontinuation in older adults. Adverse events considered for general adults apply to older adults to the extent that trials and studies include older participants. For most meta-analyses, however, participant-level descriptive data were not available; one FDA review[124,125] reported age-related results. For cohort studies, patients over 65 years were in the included age ranges, but data were not reported separately for this age group. Below we summarize available subgroup analyses from the trials and studies discussed above and summarize. One systematic review reporting on serious medical issues (upper gastrointestinal bleeding) in adults and older adults with antidepressant use.

**Suicidality:** Older patients (ages 65 years or older) on antidepressant medications showed a reduction in suicidal behaviors (OR 0.06; CI: 0.01, 0.58) and in suicidality (suicide deaths, suicidal behaviors and suicidal ideation) (OR 0.39; CI: 0.18, 0.78), compared with placebo.[124,125] For all types of suicide-related events (suicide, attempts, preparatory acts, and ideation), crude rates were lower in the antidepressant-treated group than in placebo. Cohort studies did not provide more specific information on this population subgroup.

**Serious medical issues:** We found a fair-quality systematic review of six observational studies examining the risk of bleeding in antidepressant users (particularly those on SSRIs or with greater inhibition of serotonin reuptake) which reported on patients at increased risk of UGI (upper gastrointestinal) bleeding (e.g. older persons) and also examined synergistic effects with other medications that are known causes of UGI bleeding.[132] The quality of this review was limited by searching only in MEDLINE, by inadequate reporting of search results and inclusion/exclusion activities, and by lack of quality assessment of included studies. This review included four large population-based database studies evaluating UGI bleeding and two studies evaluating any abnormal bleeding. For UGI bleeding, the four studies included a total of 14,128 cases of UGI bleeding in 419,897 persons from the UK General Practice

Research database (1993-1997), province-wide health records for older adult patients in Ontario, Canada (1992-1998), population-data from Denmark (1991-1995), and the Health Improvement Network from GPs in England and Wales (1990-2003). After excluding those with previous GI bleeding (and other risk factors for GI bleeding) from Danish cases and controls, 26,005 patients aged 16 to 104 (48 percent aged 60 years or older) using antidepressants were at increased risk of hospitalizations for UGI bleeding.[135] During periods of active SSRI use, hospitalizations for UGI bleeding were 4.3 per 1000 person-years of treatment compared with never-users, with an excess risk of 3.1 per 1000 person-years. Rates were further increased in those using SSRIs and NSAIDs only (17.7 per 1000 person-years), SSRIs and low-dose aspirin (13.0 per 1000 person-years), and SSRIs with other drugs (17.0 per 1000 person-years). Risks with SSRI use were removed after termination of treatment. To a lesser extent, rates of hospitalization for UGI bleeding were also increased in adults on older (first generation) non-SSRI antidepressants both during and after treatment. The comparison cohort was not age-or sex-matched, and there could have been differences in risk of GI bleeding between users and non-users of anti-depressants that explain different rates of bleeding between the two groups. However, demonstration of no significantly increased risk during periods when antidepressant users were not taking SSRIs (specificity of effect) increases confidence in these findings.

In 317,824 older Canadian patients (all over aged 65 years) prescribed SSRIs or other antidepressants, risk of hospitalization for UGI bleeding greatly increased with age.[134] For those aged 65-70 years, rates were comparable to the Danish study (4.1 per 1000 person-years) but increased to 7.2 per 1000 person-years in those 70-75 years, 8.8 per 1000 person-years in those 75-80 years, and 12.3 per 1000 person-years in those over 80 years of age. For older patients with a history of previous GI bleeding, hospitalizations for UGI bleeding ranged from 28.6 per 1000 person-years to 40.3 per 1000 person-years (overall 33.2 per 1000 person-years), depending on how strongly the SSRI caused serotonin inhibition. The relative risks of UGI bleeding among older persons taking SSRI antidepressants were also increased in those on non-steroidal anti-inflammatory drugs (NSAIDs) (RR 2.8; CI: 2.4, 3.3), anti-coagulants (RR 2.2; CI: 1.7, 2.8), peptic ulcer treatment (RR 2.1; CI: 1.8, 2.4) and to a lesser extent, aspirin (RR 1.7; CI: 1.4, 2.0). In the UK GPRD database, only 3.1 percent of 1651 patients aged 40-79 years with UGI bleeding were current users of SSRIs, but the odds of SSRI use or of NSAID drug use were significantly increased (2-3 fold) in persons with UGI bleeding compared with age-and-sex matched controls.[133] In this report, there was a strong interaction between these two, such that the odds were increased markedly (OR 15.6; CI: 6.6, 36.6) for NSAIDS and SSRIs combined. However another general practice-based report (The Health Improvement Network) from England and Wales found no clear increase in risk of UGI bleeding in 11,261 adult cases of UGI bleeding compared with 53,156 controls for SSRIs plus NSAIDs compared with SSRIs alone.[136] Two other studies listed in the review report on risk of any abnormal bleeding. One study from the Drug Safety Research Unit in the UK using prescription event monitoring data supplied by GPs found weak evidence to support more bleeding events in the first six months among 50,150 new users of SSRIs compared to users of other psychiatric drugs or non-psychiatric drugs.[153] As with many of these prescription event monitoring studies, adverse event ascertainment was limited due to a 51 percent response rate from surveyed GPs. In a nested case-control study from the Netherlands, rates of hospitalization from 1992-2000 for a primary diagnosis of any type of abnormal bleeding were 4.9 per 1000 person-years in 64,000 new users of second-generation antidepressants aged 18 and older, with higher risks linearly associated with greater degrees of inhibition of serotonin intake in antidepressants.[154]

We found one good-quality large prospective population-based community cohort study that evaluated the effect of daily SSRI use on the risk of clinical fragility fracture, bone mineral density, and falls over 5 years among 5008 subjects (137 daily SSRI users) aged 50 years and older.[155] After adjustment for potential confounders including age, total hip BMD, modified Charlson index, prevalent vertebral deformity, prevalent fragility fractures at baseline, and cumulative lifetime estrogen use in women, daily SSRI use was associated with a two-fold increased risk of radiographically-confirmed fragility fractures (HR 2.1, CI: 1.3, 3.4) and a reduction in bone mineral density at the total hip. In those with daily use compared with non-users, after adjustment for history of falls, there was a two-fold increased risk of falls (HR 2.2, CI: 1.4, 3.5). Fracture rates did not appear to be moderated completely by the impact of daily SSRIs on falls or on BMD, as they remained elevated after adjustments for these risk factors. The duration of use among daily SSRI users could not be confirmed.

**Tolerability:** Crude rates of early discontinuation for any reason, and for adverse effects, appeared higher in older adult patients than in younger patients. In two comparative effectiveness meta-analyses, about one-third (32 to 36 percent) of patients 55 years and older discontinued antidepressants within 3 months.[90,94] Discontinuation due to adverse effects occurred in 17 to 22 percent of seniors in clinical trials. These are unadjusted rates and are based on relatively small numbers of patients, so absolute rates should be taken as an approximation and any apparent differences may not be statistically significant.

# Summary of Evidence Quality

Table 10 summarizes the overall quality of evidence according to USPSTF criteria and other considerations about the body of evidence for each of the key questions addressed in this review.

# Chapter 4. Discussion

## Benefits and Harms of Primary Care Depression Screening

The direct evidence in support of widespread depression screening programs in primary care without further care supports beyond those focused on boosting the effectiveness of the primary care clinician's treatment is weak. However, screening programs in which other staff provide some depression care can reduce depressive symptoms. Specifically, in this review, programs in which other staff provided assessment and monitoring in coordination with the primary care provider's treatment, or that made extra efforts to enroll patients in specialty mental health treatment were likely to be effective.

We located one fair-quality RCT[10] that comparing screened and unscreened primary care adult patients; screening increased the likelihood of complete remission at three months among those with major depression, but differences were not seen in the proportion of screened and unscreened participants meeting diagnostic criteria for major depression. Methodological limitations to the analyses of interest to this review included very short follow-up, no information on the baseline comparability between the treatment and control groups in the subset of participants selected for follow-up, and no information on the comparability of the subgroup selected for follow-up with the full sample. Since only one trial directly evaluated a screening program, we also considered trials of screen-detected depressed patients, where the intervention included feedback of screening test results to clinicians (usually with provision of depression diagnostic and care management supports) compared with "usual care" where screening results were not given to the providers. The only RCT that evaluated clinician feedback of depression screening test results without further care supports (most closely mimicking a trial of screened versus unscreened patients) was a small, underpowered study that found no benefit.[113]

Feedback of screening results combined with the participation of other staff in the treatment of the patient's depression did improve depressive symptomatology,[109,110,114,116] particularly for adult patients with newly detected depression. The most intensive programs[109,110] involved extensive training of clinician and office support staff, patient materials, mental health or support staff participation in ongoing depression care, and multiple follow-up contacts. Even with a fairly intensive program, one of these trials[109] improved depression symptomatology only in patients with newly identified depression. Two less intensive programs[114,116] were also effective in reducing depressive symptomatology, when additional staff were involved in the care of the patient's depression. However, one[116] of these resulted in only a one-point difference in improvement on a 30-point depression scale, which may not reflect a clinically important difference. Participants in these two less intensive programs that improved depressive symptomatology were highly selected and not broadly representative of general primary care populations.

**Comparisons with other reviews of depression screening**. In contrast to the 2002 systematic review,[71] on which the USPSTF based it depression screening recommendation, a 2005 Cochrane review that excluded all studies including "complex quality improvement/care management" strategies, concluded that screening programs were not effective in improving health outcomes. Our findings both confirm and extend these two previous reviews. Consistent with both the USPSTF and Cochrane reviews, the limited evidence we found on screening and feedback without further care supports suggested this approach is unlikely to have an impact. We concur with the previous USPSTF review that depression care support programs including screening can improve depression symptomatology and remission in adult populations, and we are clearer about the types of effective support. Any apparent differences in the conclusions between these three reviews can largely be explained by the differences in the trials each included, as detailed in Appendix E Table 1.

**Why screening programs alone may not be effective**. It is puzzling, at first glance, why screening and feedback of results alone would not clearly improve depression outcomes, since it is fairly well-established that they do increase recognition of depression.[108] Critics of widespread depression screening suggest that the differences between clinically-detected and screen-detected cases could partially explain this discrepancy.[156,157] Patients whose depression is undetected in primary care (and would therefore only be identified through screening) tend to be less impaired and have milder levels of depression than those who are identified without screening.[9,47,49,158] Treatments such as antidepressants may have only a small effect in patients with mild depression.[159] Given this, treatment may not be initiated for patients screening positive for mild depression, as was the case in a study that used the PRIME-MD screening tool in VA outpatient medical clinics, where clinical nurse specialists disagreed with the screening diagnosis in 40 percent of the positive screening cases and therefore did not initiate antidepressant treatment.[160] Studies have also found that the patients whose depression was missed by providers had negative attitudes about antidepressants[161] and were more likely to consider their depressed mood to be due to normal fluctuations or physical causes.[162] Thus, the patients whose depression is undetected may be less likely to accept the treatment that the provider would most likely offer. Given these considerations, NICE guidelines suggest avoiding antidepressants and psychological therapies as an initial treatment in mild depression, offering strategies such as watchful waiting, advice on sleep and anxiety management, exercise, or guided self-help programs[57] as initial steps.

Another reason that screening programs alone may not be effective is that many depression cases identified will already be known to the clinician. In the trials we reviewed, about 40 to 80 percent of non-older adults screening positive were already being treated (i.e., at the time of screening or very recently).[113,114,163] Similarly, in the Seattle, WA site of an international, naturalistic study of depression treatment in primary care, 34 percent of patients screened positive on the CES-D, and 44 percent of these had been treated for depression during the previous 3 months.[164] Similarly, 51 percent of those identified using the PRIME-MD screening tool in a 1995 study were already on antidepressants.[165] The identification of such a large proportion of already identified, but untreated or under-treated, depression patients in screening programs may be one reason why ongoing depression care management and treatment options— such as counseling and mental health referrals—appear necessary to gain health benefits in screening unselected adult populations. In essence, these screening programs are providing the additional monitoring and needed supports to effectively treat depression patients in primary care.

**Comparison with reviews of depression care management interventions.** Since most of the screening studies we reviewed involved additional depression care supports, we also examined recent systematic reviews on the effectiveness of depression care management interventions for improving depression in primary care settings. Four meta-analyses looked at the effectiveness of disease management or collaborative care programs and found them generally effective,[166-169] and cost-effective.[170] Additional publications have attempted to determine particular components of effective programs.[101,171-173] All of these authors identified several care components as effective: 1) care management by a nonphysician working with the primary care physician (sometimes referred to as case management); and 2) collaborative care between physicians and mental health clinicians.[101,171-173] Solberg enumerated two additional effective components: 1) education and support of patients for self-management, and 2) attention to patient preferences.[171] These program components are generally consistent with the depression care supports we found to be part of successful screening programs in this review. Programs that did not have an effect on depression remission tended to be less intensive initiatives that did not include additional staff directly supporting patient care.[101]

Although none of these reviewers of depression care management programs identified screening as a necessary or important component, it still bears examination. A 2006 editorial identified 10 trials of depression management programs published since 1995[173] and identified common components of the programs, such as whether they employed case management, whether they identified patients through screening, and the level of involvement of specialty mental health providers in the care of the patients. We used this model, expanding the table to include two other dimensions of potential importance identified in this review: whether the trial focused on newly-identified cases of depression and whether the trial targeted older adults. We expanded the table to include additional studies that were identified in any of the reviews described above,[101,166-169] or included in the current review which addressed outpatient depression management components beyond clinician information or education and were without obvious quality concerns (Table 11). Effective trials, shown on the top half of the table, are those in which a significant treatment effect was seen at some time point for at least one of the main depression outcomes of interest. The ineffective trials are listed in the bottom section of the table and did not show significant treatment effects.

One of the most striking differences between the effective and ineffective programs was that 96 percent of the successful programs involved some kind of case or care management, compared to only 39 percent of the unsuccessful programs. One important benefit of case management is the ability to closely monitor symptoms and side effects, which in turn can help guide the depression management.[53] Also, 77 percent of the successful programs had medium-to-high levels of mental health specialist involvement, compared to only 9 percent of the unsuccessful programs. Regarding screening, 70 percent of the successful programs involved systematic screening and 39 percent of the unsuccessful programs involved screening. The data are more sparse, but just as striking, for studies focusing on older adults. All six of the successful programs targeting older adults employed case management while only two of the five (40 percent) unsuccessful programs did. All five of the successful programs reporting on mental health specialty involvement also had medium to high levels of mental health specialty care involvement, while only one (20 percent) of the unsuccessful programs did. All of the successful, and all but one of the unsuccessful, programs employed systematic screening. So, while successful programs appear more likely to have a screening component than unsuccessful programs, other components showed more striking differences between the successful and unsuccessful programs. Thus, from this exploratory analysis, it appears that while screening may be useful to such programs, other components may be more critical to the success of depression management programs.

**Harms of screening.** No evidence was found that screening for depression is harmful. Theoretical harms include any stigma or distress associated with labeling, false positives, and identifying many more cases of mild, potentially transient depression. This could increase the risk of overuse of antidepressants and create unnecessary patient costs and potential side effects, as well as unnecessary societal or health system costs. Because effective screening would likely increase the number of depressed patients using antidepressants, the probability of serious adverse events associated with antidepressant use should also be weighed carefully against their potential benefits.

**Cost-effectiveness.** A cost-effectiveness study of a primary care depression care management intervention including a one-time screening component (which was included in our review)[174] found that the intervention was cost-effective in patients who had not been previously identified as depressed. They estimated the incremental cost effectiveness ratio for enhanced care compared to usual care ranged from $9,592 to $14,306 per QALY over the course of two years.[174] However, this intervention was not continued after the trial ended, despite its promising results, raising doubts about the feasibility of this program without other facilitating factors that were present when the studied was conducted.

## Effectiveness of Depression Treatment in Older Adults

Both antidepressants and psychotherapy appear to be effective in treating depression in older adults. Two good-quality meta-analyses[120,121] published in 2000 and 2006 concluded that antidepressants are effective in treating depression in older adults, with estimated OR of 1.96 (CI: 1.39, 2.78) for SSRIs and 1.92 (CI: 1.07, 3.45) for other second generation antidepressants, compared with placebo controls. The Cochrane review published in 2000 reported 28 to 50 percent of older adults randomized to antidepressant treatment recover from depression compared with 10 to 25 percent in the placebo control groups. These recovery rates appear to be comparable to recovery rates in general adult samples: recent primary care treatment effectiveness data in adults suggests that roughly 25 to 30 percent are likely to achieve full remission and an additional 15 to 30 percent would show a response to treatment over the course of 3-6 months.[53,79] Additionally, two good-quality meta-analyses[120,122] concluded that psychotherapy is effective in treating depression in older adults. In these studies, depressed older adults were more than twice as likely to achieve remission than those who were not treated, with the ORs estimated at 2.47 (CI: 1.76, 3.47) and 2.63 (CI: 1.96, 3.53). Effect sizes estimates range from 0.72 to 1.09.

Although antidepressants and psychotherapy are effective in treating depression in older adults, most of these trials involved relatively healthy patients with mild-to-moderate levels of depressive symptomatology. Many older depressed patients may have significant challenges, including medical co-morbidities, that affect the generalizability of this research. The use of depression care management interventions, particularly psychosocial treatments, could be important to achieving real-world benefits in older and younger adults.[175] Primary care-based collaborative care approaches such as those tested by the PROSPECT and IMPACT trials, involving treatment teams including primary care clinician, depression care manager, and a mental health specialist, have improved depression outcomes and functioning in depressed older adults, with persistent benefits at up to 2 years.[176,177] The IMPACT intervention was also found to be cost-effective.[178] Considered as a whole, data on depression care management programs suggest a potential benefit for depressed patients of all ages and support calls for better links between process measures for quality care in depression, such as HEDIS, and health outcomes.[179]

## Treatment-Associated Harms in Adults and Older Adults

Controversy has existed about whether antidepressants aggravate suicide risk beginning with the use of tricyclic antidepressants (TCAs) and continuing through the introduction of second-generation antidepressants, particularly SSRIs. The proposed mechanism of action is reduction of psychomotor retardation before affect improvement and perhaps inducement of akathisia, which has been associated with increased suicidality, and which has been reported in up to 25 percent of SSRIs users early in SSRI treatment.[180] Treatment effects can be hard to determine, however, since suicidal ideation itself is a common feature of depressive disorders, occurring in 50 to 60 percent of those with MDD.[57]

We found no definitive evidence from seven separate exhaustive meta-analyses of short-term, placebo-controlled trials that second-generation antidepressants (primarily SSRIs) increase the risk of completed suicide in adults. While reassuring, these results are not conclusive, given the power limitations to detect such a rare event. Others have noted elsewhere that, given these rare event rates, 300,000 persons would need to be studied to have the power to detect a two-fold difference in suicide deaths.[129] When we calculated absolute risk differences for suicide in MDD patients treated with SSRIs or placebos, the risk differences were modest (1.12 and 1.8 per 10,000 persons treated), with 95 percent confidence intervals that crossed zero (Table 9). Thus, these results are most accurately considered consistent with some increase in short-term risk, a mild protective effect, or no increased risk for suicide in patients with MDD treated with SSRIs. Longer-term observational studies did not suggest markedly different rates of suicide over six or more months after antidepressant treatment initiation than most meta-analyses of shorter term trials, and one observational study suggested a similar rate of suicide-related deaths across the first six months of treatment;[129] both of these findings provide some reassurance that the shorter-term clinical trials are not providing drastic underestimates of suicide-related risk due to patient selection or other factors.

Meta-analyses also suggested no increase in non-fatal suicide attempts or serious self-harm behaviors, except in three analyses of adults treated with SSRIs or other second-generation antidepressants. In a careful meta-analysis conducted by the manufacturer that utilized independent, adverse event assignment by experts, definitive suicidal behavior (all events consisting of suicide attempts with no completed events or preparatory acts) was increased (OR 6.7; CI: 1.10, 149.40) in 3455 adults with MDD on paroxetine compared with 1978 on placebo-treatment. The absolute risk difference was 26.8 non-fatal suicide attempts or serious self-harm behaviors per 10,000 person treated with paroxetine (Table 9). The estimated NNT-H is 373 (CI: 208, 1818). Although this analysis included all adults with MDD, the risk was driven by young adults (18 to 30 years) in which eight of 11 events occurred. At the time these data were released, the manufacturer stated that the company "believes that young adults, particularly those with MDD, may be at increased risk for suicidal behavior during treatment with paroxetine" and recommended that labeling amendments should be undertaken.[131] In two other meta-analyses, odds of suicidal behaviors were doubled (OR 2.70, CI: 1.22, 6.97) in a meta-analysis of 10,557 adults being treated for all indications on SSRIs compared with 7856 adults on placebo[130] and in a 2006 FDA analysis restricted to young adults (18 to 24 years) being treated with second-generation antidepressants, including SSRIs, for any psychiatric indication (OR 2.31; CI: 1.02, 5.64, treatment vs. placebo-control).[125]

Any risks of self-harm that may be associated with second-generation antidepressant use are strongly age-related. In older adults (ages 65 and older), antidepressant use was protective for all suicide-related events in the FDA 2006 meta-analysis looking across the lifespan. Other studies outside the scope of this review (since absolute risks could not be assessed and/or the focus was a high-risk group) generally confirm a beneficial impact of antidepressants on suicides in older adults. Juurlink and colleagues conducted a nested case-control study using linked population-based coroners' records, patient-level prescription data, physician billing claims, and hospitalization data on 1,264,686 Ontario residents 66 years of age and older from 1992 to 2000.[181] While there was a small increased risk of suicide only during the first month of SSRI therapy compared with other antidepressants (after propensity-score adjustment for measured confounders), the absolute risk for suicide among treated patients was very low and the majority (68 percent) of older persons committing suicide had received no antidepressant therapy during the six months prior to death. In 101 Israeli older adults with MDD hospitalized for suicide attempts, fewer (42 percent) were exposed to antidepressants prior to their suicide attempt than matched controls of patients with MDD admitted to the hospital who had not attempted suicide (52 percent on antidepressants, p=0.02).[182] Some recent observational studies reviewed by others that did not meet our inclusion criteria (by reporting only relative as opposed to absolute suicide-related risks in a comparative effectiveness study) confirm findings about timing of the greatest suicide-related risks. A matched case-control study of patients treated with antidepressants in UK general practices from 1993-1999 suggests that odds of suicidal behaviors are increased during the first month (particularly the first 1 to 9 days) after a new antidepressant prescription.[148] These findings coincide with those from a large prospective cohort study in the US reviewed here.[129]

We did not generally emphasize findings for suicidal ideation combined with behaviors, as attempts and ideation appear to be distinctly affected. Nor did we include evaluations focused on individual drugs nor comparisons between drugs since most of these involve indirect comparisons (i.e., comparisons using different populations from different RCTs to supply treatment and comparison). However, we made an exception by reporting findings from the paroxetine RCTs separately due to the quality of the recent GSK analysis using blinded, expert event classification which indicated increased risk of suicide attempts in young adults, particularly those with MDD, and due to a consistent pattern of increased risk (significant or not) with paroxetine in drug-specific analyses in the most recent FDA review.[125] While small numbers of events make actual estimates of increased risk unstable, these findings are certainly worthy of current clinical attention and future research.

A puzzling finding was the discrepancies between the 2006 FDA report compared with findings from multiple other reviews, including an earlier FDA report. A more detailed consideration of these issues is included in Appendix G Table 4 "Quality concerns/Comments" column and Appendix G Table 9.

The support for care and close monitoring suggested for effective depression screening and management program in this report may also reduce potential harms. In older adults, the PROSPECT (Prevention of Suicide in Primary Care Elderly) trial found that suicidal ideation and depression severity were more effectively reduced and remission achieved more commonly in patients receiving treatment management using practice-based depression care managers than in those receiving usual care.[183] While careful monitoring of patients, particularly younger patients, during early treatment with antidepressants seems prudent, screening for suicidality would be a more direct means of detecting those at risk of suicide and has been addressed in a separate report for the USPSTF.[184] Among clinically depressed primary care patients in need of treatment, a small proportion 0.5 percent are at high risk of suicide, while about 10 percent have active thoughts but no clear plans.[185] This supports the idea that there may be high-risk groups, which could be an important area for future review by the USPSTF.

In looking for increased medical risks associated with antidepressant use in older adults, we found evidence that risks of UGI bleeding may be increased about two-to-three fold in adults currently using SSRIs, particularly older adults, those with a history of GI bleeding, and those on SSRIs with higher degrees of serotonin reuptake inhibition. Concurrent use of NSAIDs, and to a lesser extent low-dose aspirin and other anticoagulants, appeared to further increase bleeding risks. These findings may have implications for all adults, but particularly for vulnerable older adults or those with a history of GI bleeding, given the prevalence of use of analgesic medications (over-the-counter as well as prescription) for therapeutic and preventive reasons. Recent reports of a small but significant two-fold increase in falls and fractures with SSRI use in adults 50 years and older[155] suggest that clinicians should remain aware of new research about the risk-benefit ratio for different medication classes as they consider appropriate antidepressant treatment choices, particularly in older adults.

Relatively large numbers of patients discontinued therapy (16 to 29 percent) with longer-term discontinuation in community-based trials similar to population-based studies. The high rates of discontinuation in clinical trials would be reduced in actual primary care using medication counseling (not just handouts)[106] or care management interventions, which include frequent contacts to titrate medications, monitor symptoms, and address adverse effects.[75] Discontinuation due to adverse events (5 to 12 percent) might be somewhat amenable to these approaches.

# Limitations of the Review and the Literature

We limited questions of harms of treatment to existing systematic reviews, meta-analyses, and large prospective observational studies examine harms of antidepressants. We examined a limited set of pre-specified rare but serious adverse effects and also examined discontinuations (total and due to adverse events) to represent less severe, more common adverse events for all adults. For older adults, we considered a broader range of serious adverse events (serious medical events such as GI bleeding). We took this approach given the overall purpose of the report which was to provide data to estimate overall benefits and harms from screening (and subsequent treatments) for depression. Also, this approach was necessary given the very large body of international evidence on second-generation antidepressants and on depression in general. Our approach, however, omitted information from trials of more recently approved medications (e.g., duloxetine) and would not have captured rare or emerging serious medical effects that are not already well summarized in the literature or studied in large observational studies. None of the abstracts and individual papers reviewed for inclusion in this review suggested that our approach led to significant omissions.

Given that commonly available antidepressants have comparable efficacy in the majority of patients seen in primary care,[57,92] clinicians may select medications based on the consequences of specific adverse effects for individual patients (for example, dizziness in an older adult with poor balance or nausea in a patient with dyspepsia).[75] Detailed considerations of potential side effect differences were beyond the scope of this report but are considered elsewhere.[57,92]

Much of the evidence for serious suicide-related harms derives from short-term RCTs conducted for drug development and submitted to regulatory agencies. This evidence may not be generalizable to primary care due to exclusion of the most severe (or suicidal) patients, high dropout rates (which can be due to a host of factors, including withdrawal by a concerned clinician),[57] recruitment strategies outside of health care settings that tend to get motivated patients, sponsorship by the drug industry (which have been shown to be more likely to demonstrate positive effects than independent studies).[142] Also, high placebo effects are seen in some trials, and may be due to a host of factors, including the trend towards less severely depressed patients in more recent clinical trials and the ameliorating effect on depression of the support from being in a trial.[180] The very large body of evidence from hundreds of small studies makes quality review, including careful checking for completeness and systematic inclusion across reviews impossible, and undoubtedly resulted in data from some trials being included more than once, particularly across reviews. We did not attempt to summarize data between meta-analyses due to the potential for duplication as well as difference in methods.

Many reports attempt to determine the comparative harm of medications, particularly related to suicide events. Limitations of this literature are lack of a true control in a condition with increased suicide risk on its own, use of indirect comparisons, and serious concerns from confounding by indication in non-randomized comparisons, which makes it difficult to interpret results reporting either differences or similarities between medications. Jick et al, for example, found that medication differences in suicidal events were largely due to confounding by indication in a case-control analysis of 143 suicide cases and 1000 randomly selected antidepressant users from the large UK General Practice Research Database. Differences in suicide risk were no longer present after controlling for history of suicidality and number of previous antidepressant treatment episodes.[127] Others have also demonstrated confounding by indication in observational studies of suicidality and antidepressant use.[150]

We did not consider ecologic data on suicidality, as many other reviewers have, since it does not meet minimum USPSTF criteria for study designs that indicate causality. However, US data indicating a decrease in the suicide rate signal from 1988 to 2002 (after being stable from 1960-1988), during the same time fluoxetine prescriptions increased 15-fold, are consistent with no increased risk due to second generation antidepressants, an increased risk of suicidal behaviors (such as attempts) but not suicide, or increased suicide risk only with specific antidepressants or in specific subgroups (such as younger age).[186]

Our review did not include questions examining a high-risk approach to screening (e.g., screening or treatment results focused specifically on high-risk groups, such as those with a history of depression, coronary artery disease, or other medical conditions). NICE has recommended screening for depression in primary care and general hospital settings only for those in high-risk groups, but these recommendations were based on consensus rather than on evidence.[57] The presence of medical and psychiatric co-morbidities may affect depression outcomes, but we did not examine this question.

Little data were available to specifically examine the impact of race/ethnicity in depression screening or treatment. However, a pooled analysis of 104 paroxetine trials in 14,875 adults with all indications was undertaken to specifically examine response and tolerability in minority populations (Hispanic, Asians, African Americans). This study reported no treatment by minority group interaction for depressed patients, and a similar speed or response and adverse effects across groups.[187] Authors note very low power to detect differences due to the low number of minorities recruited as subjects in these studies, and suggest much greater effort to ensure minority representation in future clinical trials.

Another limitation of our review is the narrow scope of the question of efficacy of depression treatment in older adults (KQ3), for treatments we judged to be widely available to primary care providers, and in samples that are similarly to general primary care populations. Most of these data were limited to short-term treatment efficacy trials, and therefore the long-term treatment effectiveness is unknown, as is the effectiveness of these treatments in general primary care populations, as generally delivered in primary care.

For the purposes of this review, we sought to answer the focused question of whether commonly available treatments can improve depression in older adults. Therefore, we did not review trials examining the best way to deliver treatment to older adults, such as trials examining collaborative care approaches. We also excluded trials that compared different treatment agents with each other, as these did not address the focused question of whether there are efficacious treatment agents for this group of adults. We also excluded trials of physical treatments, such as ECT and TMS, as we felt these may not be widely available for referral from primary care. Finally, we also excluded trials that were limited to older adults with specific medical conditions, such as those who had recently suffered a stroke or myocardial infarction because these samples were not broadly representative of primary care the population.

Studies addressing maintenance and relapse prevention were beyond the scope of this review, but are an important area of research for clinicians.

# Future Research

Large-scale, randomized controlled trials, or at least well-controlled clinical trials of depression screening programs with an unscreened control group and health outcome ascertainment (including response, remission, and health risks), would be very useful in answering the role of depression screening in improving overall depression care management.

Better understanding of the necessary and sufficient components of depression care management programs (screening; frequency of monitoring; type of monitoring; training of monitors; role of physicians and non-physician providers, etc) that are directly relevant to improving depression outcomes in primary care would help clarify the key parts of such program.

Updated information on the frequency that depression cases are missed in current primary care, and their level of severity (e.g., major depressive disorder, dysthymia, minor depression) would help determine the current need for active case finding approaches. Consideration of how such under-diagnosis varies between different primary care settings would be key.

Better understanding of other high-risk groups for suicidal behavior and self-harm beyond young age and disease severity (MDD) would be very beneficial. Other work, for example, suggests that treatment failure may be related to underlying bipolar disorder.[188]

Better understanding of suicide and self-harm risks in various subgroups according to medication response and adverse effects (e.g., nonresponders vs. responders) could help target suicide prevention efforts. The FDA's report found results for suicidal behavior that were consistent with the increased risk occurring primarily in those who do not show a clinical response to treatment.[124,125]

Pharmacogenetic studies, such as information on metabolizer genotypes (e.g., CYP2D6), and the impact of genetic variability and of medication interactions on antidepressant efficacy, tolerability, and safety could help in targeting depression treatments to increase benefits and reduce adverse effects.[57,151]

Better understanding of the impact of depression care management programs on adverse effects and harms would help determine net benefit of these approaches.

Further understanding of risks associated with long-term antidepressant use, particularly among older adults and those taking other medications, is greatly needed.

# Conclusions

Good evidence supports the health benefits of programs combining depression screening and feedback with the support of additional staff to provide some depression care in adults visiting primary care. However, it is unclear that screening itself is a necessary part of such a program, and available evidence does not support screening alone in the absence of additional staff providing case management or mental health treatment functions. Variability among primary care settings in the rates of under-detection may further confuse one's understanding of the role of screening. The most comprehensive programs included clinician training and treatment protocols provided at the point of care, patient educational materials, office staff training and participation in providing post-visit follow-up, and available mental health referral; the mechanisms by which these interventions produce benefits are likely multiple, but could include enhanced treatment adherence through closer monitoring of treatment tolerability and response, treatment adjustments, and psychosocial support. Closer monitoring may also be important for reducing uncommon, but potentially serious, adverse events. Depression screening and feedback without additional staff to provide some of the depression care are unlikely to offer additional benefits above usual care.

Older adults benefit from antidepressants and/or psychotherapy comparable to (or almost as well as) younger adults. Older depressed adults have a reduced risk of suicide-related adverse events (ideation or behaviors) during antidepressant treatment, in contrast with younger patients. However, risks for upper gastrointestinal (UGI) bleeding, a serious medical side-effect, may be elevated at least two-to-three-fold in older patients on SSRI antidepressants, particularly in those with a history of UGI bleeding or concurrent use of NSAIDs. Antidepressants with more potent serotonin-uptake inhibition may further increase risk.

These findings may have relevance for all adults, particularly older adults, given the prevalence of SSRI, NSAID, and low-dose aspirin use.

Concerns about rare, but very serious suicide-related antidepressant treatment harms with the potential for significant public health harm due to widespread antidepressant use, have prompted repeated meta-analyses. The most current evidence on completed suicide does not demonstrate an effect of second-generation antidepressants compared with placebo, but is also consistent with mild protection or some increased risk. Although results for suicidal behavior and ideation are similar for the most part, several meta-analyses suggest a true short-term increase in suicidal behavior in young adults (aged 18-29 years) on antidepressants, particularly those with major depressive disorder and those taking paroxetine. Thus careful monitoring during early treatment, particularly in younger adults, seems prudent.

# Tables

# Table 1. Primary DSM-IV depression disorders, criteria for adults[2]

| Depressive Diagnoses | Symptoms |
|---|---|
| **Major Depressive Episode:**<br>- 5 or more depressive symptoms for $\geq$ 2 weeks<br>- Must have either depressed mood or loss of interest/pleasure<br>- Symptoms must cause significant distress or impairment<br>- No manic or hypomanic behavior<br><br>**Minor Depressive Episode:**[*]<br>- 2-4 depressive symptoms for $\geq$ 2 weeks<br>- Must have either depressed mood or loss of interest or pleasure<br>- Symptoms must cause significant distress or impairment<br>- No manic or hypomanic behavior | 1. Depressed Mood<br>2. Markedly diminished interest or pleasure in most or all activities<br>3. Significant weight loss (or poor appetite) or weight gain<br>4. Insomnia or hypersomnia<br>5. Psychomotor retardation<br>6. Fatigue or loss of energy<br>7. Feelings of worthlessness or excessive or inappropriate guilt<br>8. Diminished ability to think or concentrate, or indecisiveness<br>9. Recurrent thoughts of death (not just fear of dying), or suicidal ideation, plan, or attempt |
| **Dysthymic Disorder**<br>- Depressed mood for most of the time for at least two years<br>- Presence of 2 or more of symptoms of dysthymia<br>- Never without symptoms for 2 months or more over 2 year period<br>- Symptoms must cause clinically significant distress or impairment<br>- No major depressive disorder in first two years, no manic, hypomanic, or mixed episodes. | 1. Significant weight loss (or poor appetite) or weight gain<br>2. Insomnia or hypersomnia<br>3. Fatigue or loss of energy<br>4. Low self-esteem<br>5. Diminished ability to think or concentrate, or indecisiveness<br>6. Feelings of hopelessness |

---

[*] not a formal diagnosis but considered a research category requiring further study

# Table 2. List of antidepressants and their categorizations

| Category | Drug Class | Generic names |
|---|---|---|
| Second-generation | Selective Serotonin Re-uptake inhibitors (SSRIs) | Fluoxetine, Fluvoxamine, Paroxetine, Sertraline, Citalopram, Escitalopram |
| Second-generation | Selective Norephinephrine Re-uptake inhibitors | Venlafaxine, Mirtazapine, Duloxetine |
| Second-generation | 5-HT2 receptor antagonists | Nefazodone |
| Second-generation | Dopamine re-uptake inhibitors | Bupropion |
| First-generation | Tricyclic antidepressants (TCAs) | Amitriptyline, Clomipramine, Desipramine, Doxepin, Imipramine, Nortriptyline, Amoxapine, Protriptyline, Trimipramine |
| First-generation | Monoamine oxidase inhibitors (MAOIs) | Tranylcypromine, Phenelzine, Selegiline, Isocarboxazid |

# Table 3. Summary of results for key question 1: study examining health outcomes of a screening program in a primary care setting[10]

| | Screened (N=587) | Unscreened (N=276) | Significance |
|---|---|---|---|
| Percent female | 71% | 71% | NS |
| Mean age | 59 | 56 | NS |
| Percent Hispanic | 60% | 58% | NS |
| Annual income ≥ $16,800 | 24% | 24% | NS |
| Baseline depression diagnosis* | 13.1% | 13.8% | NS |
| 3-mo depression diagnosis*† | 37% (N=153) | 46% (N=65) | p=0.19 |
| 3-mo ≤ 1 depression symptom, among baseline depressed† | 48% (N=67) | 27% (N=30) | p<0.05 |
| Mean symptom count reduction from baseline, controlling for baseline depression severity† | 1.6 (N=153) ‡ | 1.5 (N=65) ‡ | p=0.21 |

NS-not significant or no p-value given

\* Included major depressive disorder, dysthymia, or minor depression

† Follow-up attempted on 230 only: all 101 patients with baseline depression diagnosis and random sample of 129 patients without depression, all from Texas site.

‡ Ns not reported directly but inferred from those provided for 3-mo depression diagnosis

# Table 4. Depression symptom rating scales and diagnostic interview tools.

| Instrument | Abbreviation | Number of items | Scoring range | Typical Cut-point |
|---|---|---|---|---|
| *Symptom Rating Scales* | | | | |
| Beck Depression Inventory | BDI | 21 | 0-63 | 11 mild |
| | | | | 17 borderline clinical |
| | | | | 21 moderate |
| | | | | 31 severe |
| Center for Epidemiological Studies Depression Screen | CESD | 20 | 0-16 | 16 |
| Geriatric Depression Scale | GDS | 30 | 0-30 | 14 |
| | GDS-15 | 15 | 0-15 | 5 |
| Hamilton Depression Rating Scale (Clinician rating tool) | HAMD | 21 | | |
| Montgomery-Asberg Depression Rating Scale (Clinician rating tool) | MADRS | 10 | 0-60 | None found |
| PRIME-MD Patient Health Questionnaire Brief | PHQ-9 | 9 | 0-27 | 5 mild |
| | | | | 10 moderate |
| | | | | 15 moderately severe |
| | | | | 20 severe |
| Primary Care Evaluation of Mental Disorders, Mood Module screening items | PRIME-MD brief screen | 2 | 0-2 | 2 |
| Composite International Diagnostic Interview, two "stem" items for depression section. | CIDI 2-item | 2 | 0-2 | 2 |
| *Diagnostic Interview Tools* | | | | |
| Composite International Diagnostic Interview | CIDI | (varies, depending on responses) | Diagnostic code | NA |
| Primary Care Evaluation of Mental Disorders, Mood Module | PRIME-MD | (varies, depending on responses) | Diagnostic code | NA |

NA-not applicable

# Table 5. Summary of results for key question 1a: studies examining health outcomes of screening results feedback among screen-identified depressed patients in primary care.

| Study setting | Approach to intervention beyond screening results feedback | Sample characteristics (N, gender, proportion of sample currently or recently treated for depression) | Length of follow-up | % depressed at follow-up *p<0.05 **p<0.01 | | | Scale score decrease from baseline *p<0.05 **p<0.01 | | |
|---|---|---|---|---|---|---|---|---|---|
| | | | | IV | UC | † | IV | UC | ‡ |
| **General adult populations** | | | | | | | | | |
| Bergus et al, 2005[113] Rural | None | N=59 Female: 67%(calc) Age: 41 (calc) 38% on meds for depression or anxiety | 10-wk 6-mo | 46% 48% (all NS) | 63% 62% | a a | 5.8 5.7 (all NS) | 5.8 5.0 | h |
| Jarjoura et al, 2004[114] Urban, indigent | Improve quality of PCP care; Logistical support for PCP; Other staff provide some dep. care | N=61 Female: 69%(calc) Age: 45 (calc) 0% currently treated | 6-mo 12-mo | — — | — — | | 7.6* 6.5* | 0* 0* | i |
| Wells et al, 2000[110] Wells et al 2004[118] Sherbourne et al[189] Multi-site, urban, rural | Improve quality of PCP care; Logistical support for PCP; Other staff provide some dep. care | N=1,356 Female: 71% Age: 44 % treated NR | 6-mo 12-mo 57-mo 24-mo | 40%**ǁ 42%** 38%IG1* 36%IG2 39%IG1 31%IG2 | 50%** 51%** 44%* 44% 34% 34% | b b b b c c | — — — — | — — — — | j |
| Rost et al, 2001[109] Rost et al, 2000[190] Multi-site, urban, rural Prev. known cases | Improve quality of PCP care; Logistical support for PCP; Other staff provide some dep. care | N=243 Female: 84%§ Age: 43§ 100% recently treated | 6-mo | — | — | | 14.5 (NS) | 11.0 | j |
| Rost et al, 2001[109] Rost et al, 2000[190] Rost et al, 2002[191] Newly identified cases | Improve quality of PCP care; Logistical support for PCP; Other staff provide some dep. care | N=189 Female: 84%§ Age: 43§ 0% recently treated | 6-mo 24-mo | 26%* — | 59% — | d — | 21.7* — | 13.5* — | j — |
| **Older Adult Population** | | | | | | | | | |
| Bosmans et al, 2006[115] Urban, the Netherlands | Improve quality of PCP care | N=145 Female: 60% Age: 65 (calc) 0% currently treated, 83% history of depression | 12-mo | 57% (NS) | 52% | e | 7.8 (NS) | 7.2 | k |
| Whooley et al, 2000[111] Urban | Improve quality of PCP care; Other staff provide some dep. care (minimally implemented) | N=331 Female: 61% Age: 76 (calc) 20% on antidepressant past 12 months | 24-mo | 42% (NS) | 50% | f | 1.8 (NS) | 2.2 | l |
| Callahan et al, 1994[112] Urban | Improve quality of PCP care; Logistical support for PCP | N=175 Female: 76% Age: 65 11.4% on antidepressant | 6-mo 9-mo | 87% (all NS) | 88% | g | — (all NS)¶ | — — | j j |

| Study setting | Approach to intervention beyond screening results feedback | Sample characteristics (N, gender, proportion of sample currently or recently treated for depression) | Length of follow-up | % depressed at follow-up *p<0.05 **p<0.01 | | | Scale score decrease from baseline *p<0.05 **p<0.01 | | |
|---|---|---|---|---|---|---|---|---|---|
| | | | | IV | UC | † | IV | UC | ‡ |
| Rubenstein et al, 2007[116] Urban VA | Logistical support for PCP; Other staff provide some dep. care | N=792 (n=206 screening positive for depression) Female: 3.2% Age: 74 % treated NR | 12-mo[⊤] | — | — | † | 3.7* | 2.7* | — |

calc-calculated: NS-not significant; IG-intervention group; NR-not reported; IG1=Psychotherapy, IG2=Medication Support
† Diagnostic Methods: a: PHQ ≥ 6; b: CIDI 2-item; c=CIDI full interview; d=CESD ≥ 15; e=PRIME-MD; f=GDS≥ 6; g=HAM-D≥ 16
‡ Scale Score Instrument: h=PHQ-9; i= BDI, standardized on control group change.; j= CESD; k= MADRS; l= GDS
§ These statistics refer to the entire study sample. Total sample=479, data presented on the 432 shown in this table.
|| Results for the two intervention groups were reported combined at 6- and 12-month follow-ups, and reported separately at 24- and 57-month follow-ups.
¶ Reported that groups did not differ at 6 or 9 months but did not provide exact scores
⊤Results only for subgroup that screened positive for depression

# Table 6. Summary of depression care support elements provided in programs of depression screening with feedback of results to providers.

| | General Populations | | | | | Older Adult Populations | | |
|---|---|---|---|---|---|---|---|---|
| | Bergus et al[113] | Jarjoura et al[114] | Wells* et al[110,118] | Rost et al[109,190,191] | Bosmans et al[115] | Whooley et al[111] | Callahan et al[112] | Rubenstein et al[116] |
| **Improve Quality of PCP Care** | | | | | | | | |
| Screening results given to provider for review | Yes | **Yes** | **Yes** | **Yes** | Yes | Yes | Yes | **Yes** |
| Provider prompted or trained in further assessment | | **Yes** | **Yes** | **Yes** | Yes | Yes | Yes | |
| Provider given generic treatment protocol and/or depression management training | | **Yes** | **Yes** | **Yes** | Yes | Yes | Yes | |
| Provider given patient-specific treatment recommendations | | | | | | | Yes | |
| **Logistical Support to PCP Provider** | | | | | | | | |
| Support or study staff provided proactive logistical help, e.g. with follow-up appointments, referrals | | **Yes** | **Yes** | **Yes** | | | Yes | **Yes** |
| **Other Staff Provide Some or Most of Depression Care** | | | | | | | | |
| Psychoeducational Classes | | | | | | Yes** | | |
| Support or study staff provided monitoring and/or case management | | | **Yes** | **Yes** | | | | **Yes** |
| Routine referral to behavioral counseling | | **Yes** | | | | | | |
| Study, mental health, or other specialty staff provided depression care or medication management | | Partial | **Yes** | | | | | **Partial** |
| **Other** | | | | | | | | |
| Financial commitment by provider's institution | | | **Yes** | | | | | |

Trials with statistically significant group differences shown in **bold**.
*Group differences were significant only for the subgroup or participants with newly identified depression
**This program offered a group psychoeducational class that only 12 percent of the intervention participants attended

Screening for Depression in Adults

# Table 7. Summary of the evidence for KQ3: treatment efficacy in older adults

| Reference | No. trials in meta-analysis (number of participants) | Years covered | Age range | Results — Remission: Odds Ratio (95% CI); Symptom Report: Effect Size (d) (95% CI) | |
|---|---|---|---|---|---|
| **Antidepressants** | | | | | |
| Pinquart et al, 2006[120] | 62 trials (N=3,951) | Through 2004 | Mean or median age ≥ 60 yrs | **Remission** 2.03 (1.67, 2.46) | **Self-Report of Symptoms,** Total: 0.62 (0.45, 0.79) |
| Antidepressant vs. placebo in depressed older adults | Subset focused on MDD: 31 trials (N=NR) | | | **Clinician Symptom Report,** Total 0.69 (0.57, 0.81) MDD-only 0.79 (0.64, 0.95) SSRI 0.48 (0.30, 0.66) | SSRIs 0.22 (0.10, 0.35) |
| Major and minor depressive disorders considered | | | | Atyp 0.72 (0.48, 0.95) TCA 0.93 (0.65, 1.21) MAOI 0.79 (0.51, 1.07) | Atyp 0.67 (0.37, 0.97) TCA 0.83 (0.46, 1.20) MAOI 0.80 (0.40, 1.19) |
| Wilson et al, 2000[121] | 17 trials (N=1,524)* | Through 1999 | ≥ 55 yrs or described as "elderly" | **Remission rates SSRI vs. Placebo:** 28% vs. 17%* 1.96 (1.39, 2.78)† | **MAOI vs. Placebo:** 41% vs. 10%* 5.88 (2.56, 14.28)† |
| Antidepressant vs. placebo in older adults | Subset focused on MDD: 8 trials (N=1,120)* | | | **Atypical vs. placebo** 42% vs. 27%* 1.92 (1.07, 3.45)† | **Community-dwelling subset only:** 36% vs. 21%* 2.13 (1.61, 2.86)† |
| Major and minor depressive conditions considered | Subset focused on community dwellers: 7 trials (N=1,070)* | | | **TCA vs. Placebo:** 49% vs. 25%* 3.12 (2.13, 4.76)† | **MDD subset only:** 36% vs. 20%* 2.27 (1.72, 2.94) (all p<0.05) |
| **Psychotherapy** | | | | | |
| Pinquart et al, 2006[120] | 32 trials (N=1,407) | Through 2004 | Mean or median age ≥ 60 yrs | **Remission:** 2.47 (1.76, 3.47) **Clinician Report** Total : 1.09 (0.91, 1.26) MDD-only 0.96 (0.69, 1.23) | **Self-Report** Total: 0.83 (0.69, 0.98) |
| | 9 trials exclusively MDD (n=NR) | | | | |
| Cuijpers et al, 2006[122] | 21 trials (N=1,937) | NR | Mean or median age ≥ 55 yrs | **Remission:** 2.63 (1.96, 3.53) **Symptom Report (Clinician- or Self-Report)** Total: 0.72 (0.59, 0.85) | |

*Calculated from Ns presented in text or summary tables.
†Odds ratio (95% confidence interval) computed by taking the reciprocal of the odds ratio of proportion not in remission reported in Wilson 2000.[121]
MDD–major depressive disorder; ES–Effect Size (d); OR–Odds Ratio; NR–Not Reported; SSRI–Selective Serotonin Reuptake Inhibitor; Atyp–atypical; TCA–Tricyclic Antidepressant; MAOI–Monoamine Oxidase Inhibitor; BDI–Beck Depression Inventory; GDS–Geriatric Depression Scale; HRSD–Hamilton Rating Scale for Depression

# Table 8. Summary of rate of suicide and related behavior or ideation.

| Study, Subgroup | Treatment Condition | Completed Suicide N (events/ persons) | Rate per 10,000 | OR, (95% CI) | Suicidal Behaviors N (events/ persons) | Rate per 10,000 | OR, 95% CI | Suicidal Behavior or Ideation N (events/ persons) | Rate per 10,000 | OR, 95% CI |
|---|---|---|---|---|---|---|---|---|---|---|
| **Systematic Reviews of Trials** | | | | | | | | | | |
| Levenson, 2006[125] Stone, 2006[124] Through 9/2006 | | | | | | | | | | |
| MDD only 162 RCTs | 2nd GenAD Placebo | 4/22,379 1/14,873 | 1.79 0.67 | 2.66* (0.26, 130.9) | - | - | - | 163/22,309 123/14,728 | 73.1 83.5 | 0.86 (0.67, 1.10) |
| All psychiatric indications 295 RCTs | 2nd GenAD Placebo | 5/39,799 2/27,309 | 1.3 0.73 | 1.72* (0.28, 18.01) | 79/39,729 49/27,164 | 19.9 18.0 | 1.11 (0.77, 1.61) | 248/39,729 196/27,164 | 62.4 72.2 | 0.84 (0.69, 1.02) |
| All psychiatric indications, Ages 18-24 years 272 RCTs | 2nd GenAD Placebo | - | - | - | 23/3,810 8/2,604 | 60.4 30.7 | **2.31 (1.02, 5.64)** | 47/3,810 21/2,604 | 123.4 80.6 | 1.55 (0.91, 2.70) |
| All psychiatric indications, Ages 25-30 years 295 RCTs | 2nd GenAD Placebo | - | - | - | - | - | 25-64 yrs | 41/5,558 27/3,772 | 73.8 71.6 | 25-64 yrs |
| All psychiatric indications, Ages 31-64 years 295 RCTs | 2nd GenAD Placebo | - | - | - | - | - | 1.03 (0.68, 1.58)** | 147/27,086 124/18,354 | 54.3 67.6 | 0.79 (0.64, 0.98)** |
| All psychiatric indications, Ages ≥65 years 233 RCTs | 2nd GenAD Placebo | - | - | - | - | - | **0.06 (0.01, 0.58)**** | 12/3,227 24/2,397 | 37.1 100.1 | 0.39 (0.18, 0.78) |
| Hammad 2006[137] Through 2000 | | | | | | | | | | |
| MDD only 207 RCTs | SSRIs only SSRI/other Placebo | 6/14,675 15/25,604 2/8,868 | 4.1 5.9 2.3 | SSRI vs Placebo: 1.81* (0.32, 18.37) SSRI+Other vs Placebo: 2.60* (0.60, 23.4) | - | - | - | - | - | - |
| Khan 2003[126] January 1985 - January 2000 | | | | | | | | | | |
| Indications not stated Number of RCTs not reported | SSRIs Placebo | 38/26,109 5/4,895 | 14.6 10.2 | 1.43* (0.56, 4.64) | - | - | - | - | - | - |
| Indications not stated Number of RCTs not reported | SSRIs Active controls | 38/26,109 34/17,273 | 14.6 19.7 | 0.74* (0.45, 1.21) | - | - | - | - | - | - |

| Study, Subgroup | Treatment Condition | Completed Suicide | | | Suicidal Behaviors | | | Suicidal Behavior or Ideation | | |
|---|---|---|---|---|---|---|---|---|---|---|
| | | N (events/persons) | Rate per 10,000 | OR, (95% CI) | N (events/persons) | Rate per 10,000 | OR, 95% CI | N (events/persons) | Rate per 10,000 | OR, 95% CI |
| **Gunnell 2005[138],Saperia 2006}[139]MHRA 2004[105] Through 2003** | | | | | | | | | | |
| All indications 439 RCTs | SSRIs Placebo | 9/23,804 7/17,022 | 3.8 4.1 | 0.85 (0.20, 3.40) | 128[†]/30,814 75[†]/21,689 | 41.5 34.6 | 1.21 (0.87, 1.83) | 97[‡]/26,882 80[‡]/18,822 | 36.1 42.5 | OR: 0.80 (0.49, 1.30) |
| **GSK 2006[131] Through December 2004** | | | | | | | | | | |
| MDD cases 19 RCTs | Paroxetine Placebo | - | - | - | 11/3,455 1/1,978 | 31.8 5.1 | **6.7 (1.10, 149.4)** | 31/3,455 11/1,978 | 89.7 55.6 | 1.3 (0.7, 2.8) |
| MDD cases, Ages 18-30 years. Number of RCTs not reported | Paroxetine Placebo | - | - | - | 8/612 0/339 | 130.7 0 | (cannot calculate) | | | |
| **Fergusson 2005[130] 1967 through June, 2003** | | | | | | | | | | |
| All indications 411 RCTs | SSRIs Placebo | 4/10,557 3/7,856 | 3.8 4.0 | 0.95 (0.24, 3.78) | 23/10,557 6/7,856[¶] | 21.8 7.6 | **2.70 (1.22, 6.97)** | - | - | - |
| **Storosum 2001[140] 1983 through 1997** | | | | | | | | | | |
| Likely MDD cases, 77 Short-term RCTs | SSRIs Placebo | 7/7,944 4/4,302 | 8.8 9.3 | 0.95* (0.24, 4.42) | 29/7,944 17/4,302 | 36.5 39.5 | 0.92* (0.49, 1.79) | - | - | - |

| Study, Subgroup | Treatment Condition | Completed Suicide | | Suicidal Behaviors | |
|---|---|---|---|---|---|
| | | N (events/ persons) | Rate per 10,000 (95% CI) | N (events/ persons) | Rate per 10,000 (95% CI) |
| Cohort Studies (includes 95% CI around event rate if no comparison) | | | | | |
| Simon 2006[129] MDD only in pre-paid group practice | Second generation and TCAs | 31/ 65,103 | 4.8 (*3.3, 6.8) | 76/ 65,103 | 11.7 (*9.3, 14.6) |
| Martinez 2005[128] Age <90 with new antidepressant prescription | Any anti-depressant (Primarily 1st generation) | 69/ 146,095 | 4.7 (*3.7, 6.0) | 1968†/ 146,095 | 134.7 (*128.9, 140.8) |
| Martinez 2005[128] 19-30 year-olds with new antidepressant prescription | Any anti-depressant (Primarily 1st generation) | 19/ 34,792 | 5.5 (*3.5, 8.6) | 747/ 34,792 | 214.7 (*199.8, 230.7) |
| Jick 1995[127] Pharmaceutical event monitoring data, All indications | Any anti-depressant (Primarily 1st generation) | 143/ 172,598 | 8.3 (*7.0, 9.8) | - | - |

Bolded: p < 0.05
*calculated
** Cited in Stone 2006
†Non-fatal harms, plus includes fluoxetine-related suicides for Gunnell.
‡Ideation only
MDD-major depressive disorder; TCA- tricyclic antidepressant; SSRI- selective serotonin reuptake inhibitor

# Table 9. Risk differences (per 10,000) for suicide and suicidality among patients with major depressive disorder.

| Study, Outcome, Comparison | Absolute Risk per 10,000, Drug | Absolute Risk, per 10,000 Placebo | Risk Difference | 95% CI |
|---|---|---|---|---|
| FDA 2006[124,125] Suicide, SSRI vs. Placebo | 1.79 (4/22379) | 0.67 (1/14873) | 1.12 | -1.1, 3.3 |
| Hammad 2006[137] Suicide, SSRI vs. Placebo | 4.1 (6/14675) | 2.3 (2/8868) | 1.8 | -2.7, 6.3 |
| GSK Report 2006[131] Suicidal Behavior, Paroxetine vs. Placebo | 31.8 (11/3455) | 5.1 (1/1978) | 26.8 | 5.5, 48.0 |
| GSK Report 2006[131] Suicidal Behavior or Ideation, Paroxetine | 89.7 (31/3455) | 55.6 (11/1978) | 34.1 | -11.3, 79.5 |

# Table 10. Summary of Evidence

| No. of studies | Design | Limitations | Consistency | Applicability | Overall Quality | Summary of Findings |
|---|---|---|---|---|---|---|
| **KQ1. Depression outcomes in screened vs. unscreened patients** | | | | | | |
| 1[10] | Controlled comparison (Subgroup analysis of larger RCT) | Single study; follow-up limited to one of two sites and to depressed patients plus random sample with depressive symptoms; not a truly randomized comparison; contamination possible. | Not applicable | Fair; representative primary care sample, but results do not represent population-level results from a screening program. | Fair | Increased likelihood of remission at 3 months among those with depression diagnosis at baseline interview (48% remission in screened vs. 27% in unscreened), but overall proportion with depression diagnoses at follow up did not differ between screened and unscreened groups (37% in screened vs. 46% in unscreened). |
| **KQ1a. Depression outcomes in trials of screening + feedback (+ other supports allowed) vs. screening without feedback** | | | | | | |
| 8[109-116] | RCTs, two randomized at the patient level; six at the clinic or practice session level; three of those using clinic-level randomization trials used cluster randomization | No non-screened control groups; considerable variability in intensity and type of additional care supports provided. | Fair; some studies found a positive effect and some did not; considerable variability on several dimensions (e.g. type of care supports, population characteristics) which may explain inconsistencies | Fair; all involved screen-detected primary care samples, although 2 limited enrollment to only those with newly detected depression and an additional trial included only patients screening positive for multiple conditions, one of which was depression, thus limiting generalizability to general primary care populations. | Fair to good; most studies fair quality, but also had two good quality large-scale trials. | Four trials of screening and feedback alone or with extra components to improve the effectiveness of the primary care provider's treatment did not improve depression at 6-12 month follow-up compared with screening without feedback in usual care. Four programs with additional staff providing depression treatment or case management to depressed patients reduced depression, though only among patients with newly-identified depression in two cases (on trial limited participants to newly-identified patients, on reported results separately for newly-identified patients). We cannot determine the degree to which screening and feedback was necessary to the programs' successes. One of the four trials in older adults was effective in improving depression, which was the only trial in older adults that included substantial involvement of staff other than primary care provider. |
| **KQ2. Harms of screening** | | | | | | |
| No evidence | | | | | | |

| Design | Limitations | Consistency | Applicability | Overall Quality | Summary of Findings |
|---|---|---|---|---|---|

**KQ3. Treatment in older adults**

| No. of studies | Design | Limitations | Consistency | Applicability | Overall Quality | Summary of Findings |
|---|---|---|---|---|---|---|
| 3[120-122] | Meta-analyses | Included trials outside the scope of our review, e.g., patients in residential or inpatient settings and studies involving minor depression. | Good | Fair; most trials very short term and not done in primary care settings; many trials only included patients with mild-moderate depression and limited comorbidities; some trials conducted in residential or inpatient settings. | Good | Antidepressants and psychotherapy are effective in treating older adult patients. Patients taking antidepressants were roughly twice as likely to achieve remission than those taking placebo pills, and patients in psychotherapeutic treatment were more than twice as likely to achieve remission than those in control conditions, which included wait-list, attention placebo, or pill placebo. |

**KQ4. Harms of antidepressant treatment in adults and older adults**

*Suicide and Suicide related events*

| No. of studies | Design | Limitations | Consistency | Applicability | Overall Quality | Summary of Findings |
|---|---|---|---|---|---|---|
| 13[125-131,137,138,140,143,144,146] | Individual and trial-level meta-analyses of placebo controlled drug efficacy RCTs in 6 regulatory reviews (and associated reports) and 1 systematic review<br><br>6 large cohort studies in US, UK, and Denmark following 1,064,603 pts for 6 months to 5 years after receiving antidepressant prescriptions | Most trials were short-term (6-8 week) efficacy trials for drug approval. Between-trial differences in outcome definitions, ascertainment time periods, and treated populations limit comparability of findings. Low event rates minimize power. | Findings across analyses are consistent for age-related differences in risks for suicide-related antidepressant treatment harms, for the timing of greatest risk for suicide-related events, and for highest risk of suicide-related events in patients with MDD and in males. Absolute event rates differ across meta-analyses more than can be explained. Cohort studies complement and extend findings from RCTs. | Fair due to RCTs including more highly selected, lower risk populations than primary care and due to short-term trial duration. Cohort studies provide additional follow-up in less selected patients treated with antidepressants through 10 months and are generally consistent with rates of suicide in clinical trials. | Fair-to-Good | Current evidence does not demonstrate an impact on suicides in those treated with second-generation antidepressants (mostly SSRIs) compared with placebo, although results are also consistent with a small protection or some increase in risk. Suicidal behaviors appear to be increased in young adults (aged 18-29), particularly those with major depressive disorder and those on paroxetine. The impact of antidepressant treatment on suicidal ideation appears to differ from the impact on suicidal behaviors, but many analyses combine these. In older adults, treatment with antidepressants confers a statistically significant protective effect on suicidal behavior and on suicidality.<br><br>In cohort studies with 6-8 month follow-up duration, crude suicide rates were 4.7 to 4.8 per 10,000 persons treated, with higher rates reported among children and adults under 30. These rates are comparable to the findings in many of the short-term RCT meta-analyses in adult groups not restricted to major depressive disorder. Men had increased risks (at least 3 times greater) for suicide deaths compared with women. In contrast, there were no sex differences in self-harm risks, and rates varied substantially between studies due to definitional (and perhaps ascertainment) differences. These studies consistently indicate the highest risk for suicidal behaviors is in the month prior to and immediately after beginning antidepressant treatment. |

| No. of studies | Design | Limitations | Consistency | Applicability | Overall Quality | Summary of Findings |
|---|---|---|---|---|---|---|

**KQ4. Harms of antidepressant treatment in adults and older adults (continued)**

*Tolerability*

| No. of studies | Design | Limitations | Consistency | Applicability | Overall Quality | Summary of Findings |
|---|---|---|---|---|---|---|
| 9[46,72,90,92-96,192] | Meta-analyses of short-term placebo-controlled RCTs in 7 systematic reviews<br><br>2 uncontrolled primary-care and specialty community-based treatment trials | Tolerability is a non-specific measure of minor but common adverse effects | Fair—differences in measurement, study durations, and populations make ranges most accurate estimates. Short-term and long-term studies generally consistent. | Fair—3 systematic reviews focused on primary care patients. Data gathered under clinical trial situations may not reflect real-world treatment experience. | Fair-to-Good | In primary care patients with depression, early antidepressant discontinuation for any reason ranges from 16% to 29%, with a best estimate of 20% to 23%. Discontinuation due to adverse events in primary care patients ranges from 5% to 12% in the first 2-3 months to 26% at nine months. In some studies, higher doses of medication and older age were associated with increased rates of early discontinuation (overall and due to adverse effects). |

*Serious medical events (upper GI bleeding)*

| No. of studies | Design | Limitations | Consistency | Applicability | Overall Quality | Summary of Findings |
|---|---|---|---|---|---|---|
| 2[132,155] | 1 qualitative systematic review of 4 large population-based studies of 419,897 adults taking antidepressants (14,128 cases of UGI bleeding)<br><br>1 large prospective cohort study | Only large observational studies were located; no trial evidence. We relied on the reviewers findings with some checking of the original articles. | Consistent findings between studies of bleeding. Specificity of effect supported by association between active SSRI use and UGI bleeds (compared with periods off drugs) and by increased risk in medications with greater serotonin reuptake inhibition. | Good | Fair-to-Good | Low-risk older patients on SSRIs had an excess risk of 3.1 UGI bleeds per 1000 treatment years during periods of active SSRI use compared with non-use and an excess of hospitalizations for UGIB of 4.1 per 1000 treatment years among older antidepressant users and 11.7 to 12.3 per 1000 treatment years in persons with prior UGI bleeding or those over 80 years of age. Increased UGI bleeds in adults 40-79 years currently taking SSRIs (adj. OR 3.0, 95% 2.1, 4.4) were much higher with concurrent use of NSAIDs (adj OR 12.2, 95% CI 7.1, 9.5) and to a lesser extent, low-dose aspirin (adj. OR 5.2, 95% CI 3.2, 8.0). To a lesser degree, UGI bleeds increased in current non-SSRI antidepressant users, (OR 1.4, 95% 1.1, 1.9) but with no interaction with NSAIDs or aspirin. UGI bleed risk associated with SSRIs showed greater increase in medications with a moderate to high degree of serotonin reuptake inhibition.<br><br>Daily SSRI use was associated with a two-fold increased risk of fragility fractures and risk of falls. |

57

Screening for Depression in Adults

# Table 11. Elements of depression management interventions[166,168,169,173,193]

| Trial | Evidence-based guideline? | Patients identified through screening? | Enhanced patient education? | Employed case mgmt? | Level of mental health specialist involvement | Newly-ID'd depression episode? [†] | Older Adult Focus? |
|---|---|---|---|---|---|---|---|
| **Effective Programs** | | | | | | | |
| Oslin 2003[194] | Yes | Yes | Yes | Yes | High | Unclear | No |
| Datto 2003[195] (pilot for Oslin) | Yes | No | Yes | Yes | High | Mix | No |
| Katon 2004[196] (Diabetes + Depression) | Yes | Yes | Yes | Yes | Medium | Mix | No |
| Bruce 2004[183] | Yes | Yes | Yes | Yes | High | Mix | Yes |
| Alexopoulis 2005[177] | Yes | Yes | Yes | Yes | Medium | Mix | Yes |
| Fortney 2006[197] | Yes | Yes | Yes | Yes | Medium | Mix | No |
| Wang 2007[198] | Yes | Yes | Yes | Yes | High | Mix | No |
| Rubenstein 2007[116] | Unclear | Yes | Unclear | Yes | Unknown | Mix | Yes |
| Unutzer 2002[199] | Yes | Yes | Yes | Yes | Medium | Mix | Yes |
| Dietrich 2004[200] | Yes | No | No | Yes | Medium | Mix | No |
| Hedrick 2003[201] | Yes | Yes | Yes | Yes | High | Mix | No |
| Rost 2001:[109,191] newly identified | Yes | Yes | Yes | Yes | Medium | Yes | No |
| Katzelnick 2000[202] | Yes | Yes | Yes | Yes | Medium | No | No |
| Hunkeler 2000 [176,203] (IMPACT) | Yes | No | Yes | Yes | Low | Yes | No |
| Wells 2000[110] | Yes | Yes | Yes | Yes | Varied | Mix | No |
| Simon 2000[204] | Yes | No | Yes | Yes | Low | Yes | No |
| Peveler 1999: Nurse counseling[205] | No | No | Yes | Yes | None | Yes | No |
| Banerjee 1996[206] | Unclear | Yes | No | Yes | High | Yes | Yes |
| Schulberg 1996:[207] IPT | No | Yes | Yes | No | High | Yes | No |
| Schulberg 1996: [207] Nortriptyline | Yes | Yes | Yes | Yes, by other physician | Low | Yes | No |
| Katon 1995, 1996[208,209] | Yes | No | Yes | Yes | High | Mix | No |
| Katon 1999[210] | Yes | No | Yes | Yes | High | No | No |
| Blanchard 1995[211] | No | Yes | No | Yes | Medium | Mix | Yes |
| *Summary* | *18/21= Yes (86%)* | *16/23=Yes (70%)* | *19/22=Yes (86%)* | *22/23=Yes (96%)* | *17/22=Med-High (77%)* | *7/22=Yes (32%)* | *6/23=Yes (26%)* |
| **Ineffective Programs** | | | | | | | |
| Ell, 2007[212] (Home Health) | Yes | Yes | Yes | Yes | High | Mix | Yes |
| Finley 2003[213] | Yes | No | Unclear | Yes | None | Yes | No |
| Swindle 2003[160] | Yes | Yes | Yes | Yes | Low | Mix | No |
| Capoccia 2004[214] | Unclear | No | Yes | Yes | None | Yes | No |
| Adler 2004[215] | Yes | Yes | Yes | Yes | None | Mix | No |
| Dobscha 2006[216] | Yes | No | Yes | No, "decision support team" | Low | Mix | No |
| Brook 2005[217] | Unclear | No | Yes | No | None | Yes (new AD) | No |
| Rollman 2002[218] | Yes | Yes | No | No | None | Mix | No |
| Rost 2001:[109] previously detected | Yes | Yes | Yes | Yes | Medium | No | No |

[†] No=only previously treated, Mix=both

| Trial | Evidence-based guideline? | Patients identified through screening? | Enhanced patient education? | Employed case mgmt? | Level of mental health specialist involvement | Newly-ID'd depression episode? [†] | Older Adult Focus? |
|---|---|---|---|---|---|---|---|
| Simon 2000:[204] Feedback only | Yes | No | Yes | No | None | Yes | No |
| Peveler 1999: Pt. Educ only[205,219] | No | No | Yes | No | None | Yes | No |
| Callahan 1994[112] | Yes | Yes | Yes | No | None | Mix | Yes |
| Dowrick 1995[220] | Yes | Yes | No | No | None | Mix | No |
| Thompson 2000[221] | Yes | No | No | No | None | Mix | No |
| Whooley 2000[111] | Unclear | Yes | Yes | No | None | Mix | Yes |
| Brown 2000:[222] Academic Detailing | Yes | No | No | No | None | Mix | No |
| Goldberg 1998:[223] Academic Detailing | Yes | No | No | No | None | Mix | No |
| Mann1998:[224] assessment + feeback | No | No | No | No | None | Mix | No |
| Mann 1998:[224] above + nurse follow-up care | No | No | No | Yes | None | Mix | No |
| Coleman 1999[225] | No | No | Yes | Yes | None | No | Yes |
| Bashir 2000[226] | Yes | No | Yes | No | None | Mix | No |
| Solberg 2001[227] | Yes | No | Yes | Yes | None | Mix | No |
| Arthur 2002[228] | No | Yes | No | No | Assessment only | No | Yes |
| Summary | 15/20= Yes (75%) | 9/23=Yes (39%) | 14/22=Yes (64%) | 9/23=Yes (39%) | 2/23=Med-High (9%) | 5/23=Yes (22%) | 5/23=Yes (22%) |

# Figures

# Figure 1. Analytic Framework

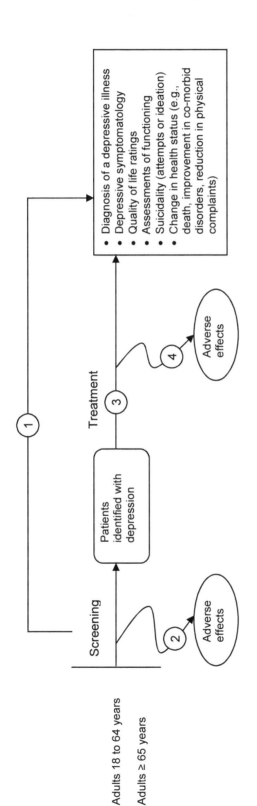

Adults 18 to 64 years

Adults ≥ 65 years

Screening

Treatment

Patients identified with depression

Adverse effects

Adverse effects

- Diagnosis of a depressive illness
- Depressive symptomatology
- Quality of life ratings
- Assessments of functioning
- Suicidality (attempts or ideation)
- Change in health status (e.g., death, improvement in co-morbid disorders, reduction in physical complaints)

1. Is there direct evidence that screening for depression among adults and the elderly in primary care reduces morbidity and/or mortality?
   a. What is the impact of clinician feedback of screening test results (with or without additional care management support) on depression response and remission in screen-detected depressed patients receiving usual care?

2. What are the adverse effects of screening for depressive disorders in adults and in elderly patients in primary care?

3. Is antidepressant and/or psychotherapy treatment of elderly depressed patients effective in improving health outcomes?

4. What are the adverse effects of antidepressant treatment (particularly SSRIs and other second-generation drugs) for depression in adults and the elderly?

# Reference List

1. Pignone M, Gaynes B, Rushton J et al. Screening for depression: A systematic review. *Agency for Healthcare Research and Quality*. 2002.

2. American Psychiatric Association. *Diagnostic and Statical Manual of Mental Disorders*. Fourth ed. Washington, DC: American Psychiatric Association. 1994.

3. Kessler RC, Chiu WT, Demler O, Merikangas KR, Walters EE. Prevalence, severity, and comorbidity of 12-month DSM-IV disorders in the National Comorbidity Survey Replication. *Arch Gen Psychiatry*. 2005;62:617-627.

4. Hasin D, Goodwin RD, Stinson F, Grant B. Epidemiology of Major Depressive Disorder: Results From the National Epidemiologic Survey on Alcoholism and Related Conditions. *Arch Gen Psychiatry*. 2005;62:1097-1106.

5. Narrow WE, Rae DS, Robins LN, Regier DA. Revised prevalence estimates of mental disorders in the United States: using a clinical significance criterion to reconcile 2 surveys' estimates. *Arch Gen Psychiatry*. 2002;59:115-123.

6. Horwath E, Cohen R, Weissman MM. Epidemiology of Depressive and Anxiety Disorders. In: Tsuang M, Tohen M, eds. *Textbook in Psychiatric epidemiology*. 2nd ed. Hoeboken, NJ: John Wiley & Sons, Inc.; 2002:389-426.

7. Beekman AT, Copeland JR, Prince MJ. Review of community prevalence of depression in later life. *Br J Psychiatry*. 1999;174:307-311.

8. Norton MC, Skoog I, Toone L et al. Three-year incidence of first-onset depressive syndrome in a population sample of older adults: the Cache County study. *Am J Geriatr Psychiatry*. 2006;14:237-245.

9. Simon GE, VonKorff M. Recognition, management, and outcomes of depression in primary care. *Arch Fam Med*. 1995;4:99-105.

10. Williams J, Mulrow CD, Kroenke K. Case-finding for depression in primary care: a randomized trial. *The American journal of medicine*. 1999;106:36-43.

11. Coyne JC, Fechner-Bates S, Schwenk TL. Prevalence, nature, and comorbidity of depressive disorders in primary care. *Gen Hosp Psychiatry*. 1994;16:267-276.

12. Spitzer RL, Williams JB, Kroenke K et al. Utility of a new procedure for diagnosing mental disorders in primary care. The PRIME-MD 1000 study. *JAMA*. 1994;272:1749-1756.

13. Lyness JM, Caine ED, King DA, Cox C, Yoediono Z. Psychiatric disorders in older primary care patients. *J Gen Intern Med*. 1999;14:249-254.

14. Schulberg HC, Mulsant B, Schulz R, Rollman BL, Houck PR, Reynolds CF, III. Characteristics and course of major depression in older primary care patients. *Int J Psychiatry Med*. 1998;28:421-436.

15. Gaynes BN, Rush AJ, Trivedi MH et al. Major depression symptoms in primary care and psychiatric care settings: a cross-sectional analysis. *Ann Fam Med*. 2007;5:126-134.

16. Gaynes BN, Rush AJ, Trivedi M et al. A direct comparison of presenting characteristics of depressed outpatients from primary vs. specialty care settings: preliminary findings from the STAR*D clinical trial. *General Hospital Psychiatry 2005 Apr. 27(2):87-96*.

17. Depression Guideline Panel. *Depression in primary care: Detection and Diagnosis. Clinical Practice Guideline: Number 5.* AHCPR Publication No. 93-0550 ed. United States Department of Health and Human Services; Public Health Service; Agency for Health Care Policy and Research; 1993.

18. Olfson M, Broadhead WE, Weissman MM et al. Subthreshold psychiatric symptoms in a primary care group practice. *Arch Gen Psychiatry*. 1996;53:880-886.

19. World Health Organization (WHO). Global Burden of Disease in 2002: data sources, methods and results. *World Health Organization (WHO)*. 2007;Global Programme on Evidence for Health Policy Discussion Paper No. 54.

20. Unutzer J, Patrick DL, Diehr P, Simon G, Grembowski D, Katon W. Quality adjusted life years in older adults with depressive symptoms and chronic medical disorders. *Int Psychogeriatr*. 2000;12:15-33.

21. Kessler RC, Berglund P, Demler O et al. The epidemiology of major depressive disorder: results from the National Comorbidity Survey Replication (NCS-R). *JAMA*. 2003;289:3095-3105.

22. Simon GE. Social and economic burden of mood disorders. *Biol Psychiatry*. 2003;54:208-215.

23. Beck CT. Maternal depression and child behaviour problems: a meta-analysis. *J Adv Nurs*. 1999;29:623-629.

24. Downey G, Coyne JC. Children of depressed parents: an integrative review. *Psychol Bull*. 1990;108:50-76.

25. Kane P, Garber J. The relations among depression in fathers, children's psychopathology, and father-child conflict: a meta-analysis. *Clin Psychol Rev*. 2004;24:339-360.

26. Penninx BW, Leveille S, Ferrucci L, van Eijk JT, Guralnik JM. Exploring the effect of depression on physical disability: longitudinal evidence from the established populations for epidemiologic studies of the elderly. *Am J Public Health.* 1999;89:1346-1352.

27. Bruce ML, Seeman TE, Merrill SS, Blazer DG. The impact of depressive symptomatology on physical disability: MacArthur Studies of Successful Aging. *Am J Public Health.* 1994;84:1796-1799.

28. Ormel J, VonKorff M, Oldehinkel AJ, Simon G, Tiemens BG, Ustun TB. Onset of disability in depressed and non-depressed primary care patients. *Psychol Med.* 1999;29:847-853.

29. Katon W, Ciechanowski P. Impact of major depression on chronic medical illness. *J Psychosom Res.* 2002;53:859-863.

30. Ferketich AK, Schwartzbaum JA, Frid DJ, Moeschberger ML. Depression as an antecedent to heart disease among women and men in the NHANES I study. National Health and Nutrition Examination Survey. *Arch Intern Med.* 2000;160:1261-1268.

31. Katon W, Russo J, Frank E et al. Predictors of nonresponse to treatment in primary care patients with dysthymia. - *General Hospital Psychiatry.* 2002;24:20-27.

32. Wulsin LR, Vaillant GE, Wells VE. A systematic review of the mortality of depression. *Psychosom Med.* 1999;61:6-17.

33. Unutzer J, Patrick DL, Marmon T, Simon GE, Katon WJ. Depressive symptoms and mortality in a prospective study of 2,558 older adults. *Am J Geriatr Psychiatry.* 2002;10:521-530.

34. McCusker J, Cole M, Ciampi A, Latimer E, Windholz S, Belzile E. Does depression in older medical inpatients predict mortality? *Journals of Gerontology Series A-Biological Sciences & Medical Sciences.* 2006;61:975-981.

35. Simon GE, VonKorff M. Suicide mortality among patients treated for depression in an insured population. *Am J Epidemiol.* 1998;147:155-160.

36. Chisholm D. The Economic Consequences of Depression. In: dawson a, Tylee A, eds. *Depression: Social and Economic Timebomb.* World Health Organization; 2001:121-9.

37. Greenberg PE, Kessler RC, Birnbaum HG et al. The economic burden of depression in the United States: how did it change between 1990 and 2000? *J Clin Psychiatry.* 2003;64:1465-1475.

38. von KL, Akerblad AC, Bengtsson F, Carlsson A, Ekselius L. Cost of depression: effect of adherence and treatment response. *Eur Psychiatry.* 2006;21:349-354.

39. Rice D, Miller L. The Economic Burden of Affective Disorder. *Br J Psychiatry.* 1995;166:34-42.

40. Pearson SD, Katzelnick DJ, Simon GE, Manning WG, Helstad CP, Henk HJ. Depression among high utilizers of medical care. *J Gen Intern Med.* 1999;14:461-468.

41. Scott J. Depression should be managed like a chronic disease. *BMJ.* 2006;332:985-986.

42. Goldberg D. The "NICE Guideline" on the treatment of depression. *Epidemiol Psichiatr Soc.* 2006;15:11-15.

43. Pincus HA, Tanielian TL, Marcus SC et al. Prescribing Trends in Psychotropic Medications: Primary Care, Psychiatry, and Other Medical Specialties. *JAMA: The Journal of the American Medical Association.* 1998;279:526-531.

44. Harman JS, Veazie PJ, Lyness JM. Primary care physician office visits for depression by older Americans. *J Gen Intern Med.* 2006;21:926-930.

45. Coryell W, Akiskal HS, Leon AC et al. The time course of nonchronic major depressive disorder. Uniformity across episodes and samples. National Institute of Mental Health Collaborative Program on the Psychobiology of Depression--Clinical Studies. *Arch Gen Psychiatry.* 1994;51:405-410.

46. Rush AJ, Trivedi MH, Wisniewski SR et al. Acute and longer-term outcomes in depressed outpatients requiring one or several treatment steps: a STAR*D report. *Am J Psychiatry.* 2006;163:1905-1917.

47. Goldberg D, Privett M, Ustun B, Simon G, Linden M. The effects of detection and treatment on the outcome of major depression in primary care: a naturalistic study in 15 cities. *Br J Gen Pract.* 1998;48:1840-1844.

48. Kessler D, Bennewith O, Lewis G, Sharp D. Detection of depression and anxiety in primary care: follow up study. *BMJ 2002 325(7371):1016-7.*

49. Thompson C, Ostler K, Peveler RC, Baker N, Kinmonth AL. Dimensional perspective on the recognition of depressive symptoms in primary care: The Hampshire Depression Project 3. *Br J Psychiatry.* 2001;179:317-323.

50. Gaynes BN, Rush AJ, Trivedi MH et al. Primary versus specialty care outcomes for depressed outpatients managed with measurement-based care: results from STAR*D. *J Gen Intern Med.* 2008;23:551-560.

51. Patten SB. A major depression prognosis calculator based on episode duration. *Clin Pract Epidemiol Ment Health.* 2006;2:13.

52. Clinical Practice and Epidemiology in Mental Health . 1-30-2007.

53. Trivedi MH, Rush AJ, Wisniewski SR et al. Evaluation of outcomes with citalopram for depression using measurement-based care in STAR*D: implications for clinical practice. *Am J Psychiatry.* 2006;163:28-40.

54. Mitchell AJ, Subramaniam H. Prognosis of depression in old age compared to middle age: a systematic review of comparative studies. *Am J Psychiatry.* 2005;162:1588-1601.

55. Cole MG, Bellavance F, Mansour A. Prognosis of depression in elderly community and primary care populations: a systematic review and meta-analysis. *Am J Psychiatry.* 1999;156:1182-1189.

56. Lyness JM, Caine ED, King DA, Conwell Y, Duberstein PR, Cox C. Depressive disorders and symptoms in older primary care patients: one-year outcomes. *Am J Geriatr Psychiatry.* 2002;10:275-282.

57. National Collaborating Centre for Mental Health. Depression: Management of Depression in Primary and Secondary Care. Clinical Guideline 23. 1-63. 2004. London, National Institute for Clinical Excellence.

58. Riolo SA, Nguyen TA, Greden JF, King CA. Prevalence of depression by race/ethnicity: findings from the National Health and Nutrition Examination Survey III. *Am J Public Health.* 2005;95:998-1000.

59. Grant BF, Stinson FS, Dawson DA et al. Prevalence and co-occurrence of substance use disorders and independent mood and anxiety disorders: results from the National Epidemiologic Survey on Alcohol and Related Conditions. *Arch Gen Psychiatry.* 2004;61:807-816.

60. Simon GE. Treating depression in patients with chronic disease: recognition and treatment are crucial; depression worsens the course of a chronic illness. *West J Med.* 2001;175:292-293.

61. Lorant V, Deliege D, Eaton W, Robert A, Philippot P, Ansseau M. Socioeconomic inequalities in depression: a meta-analysis. *Am J Epidemiol.* 2003;157:98-112.

62. Ames D. Depression and the elderly. In: Dawson A, Tylee A, eds. *Depression: Social and exonomic timebomb.* London: BMJ Publishing Group; BMA House;Tavistock Square; 2001:49-62.

63. NIH consensus conference. Diagnosis and treatment of depression in late life. *JAMA.* 1992;268:1018-1024.

64. Luoma JB, Martin CE, Pearson JL. Contact with mental health and primary care providers before suicide: a review of the evidence. *Am J Psychiatry.* 2002;159:909-916.

65. Serby M, Yu M. Overview: depression in the elderly. *Mt Sinai J Med.* 2003;70:38-44.

66. Krishnan KR, Delong M, Kraemer H et al. Comorbidity of depression with other medical diseases in the elderly. *Biol Psychiatry.* 2002;52:559-588.

67. Practice guideline for the treatment of patients with major depressive disorder (revision). American Psychiatric Association. *Am J Psychiatry.* 2000;157:1-45.

68. Rush AJ, Kraemer HC, Sackeim HA et al. Report by the ACNP Task Force on response and remission in major depressive disorder. *Neuropsychopharmacology.* 2006;31:1841-1853.

69. Judd LL, Akiskal HS, Zeller PJ et al. Psychosocial disability during the long-term course of unipolar major depressive disorder. *Arch Gen Psychiatry.* 2000;57:375-380.

70. Penninx BW, Guralnik JM, Ferrucci L, Simonsick EM, Deeg DJ, Wallace RB. Depressive symptoms and physical decline in community-dwelling older persons. *JAMA.* 1998;279:1720-1726.

71. Pignone MP, Gaynes BN, Rushton JL et al. Screening for depression in adults: a summary of the evidence for the U.S. Preventive Services Task Force. *Ann Intern Med.* 2002;136:765-776.

72. Arroll B, MacGillivray S, Ogston S et al. Efficacy and tolerability of tricyclic antidepressants and SSRIs compared with placebo for treatment of depression in primary care: a meta-analysis. *Annals of Family Medicine 3(5):449-56.* 2005;-Oct.

73. Bech P, Cialdella P, Haugh MC et al. Meta-analysis of randomised controlled trials of fluoxetine v. placebo and tricyclic antidepressants in the short-term treatment of major depression. *Br J Psychiatry.* 2000;176:421-428.

74. Geddes JR, Freemantle N, Mason J, Eccles MP, Boynton J. Selective serotonin reuptake inhibitors (SSRIs) versus other antidepressants for depression. *Cochrane Database of Systematic Reviews.* 2005.

75. Williams JW, Jr., Mulrow CD, Chiquette E, Noel PH, Aguilar C, Cornell J. A systematic review of newer pharmacotherapies for depression in adults: evidence report summary. *Ann Intern Med.* 2000;132:743-756.

76. Shah, Rajen, Uren, Z., Baker, A., and Majeed, A. Deaths from antidepressants in England and Wales 1993-1997: Analysis of a new national database. Psychological Medicine 31[7], 1203-1210. 2001.

77. Pirraglia PA, Stafford RS, Singer DE. Trends in Prescribing of Selective Serotonin Reuptake Inhibitors and Other Newer Antidepressant Agents in Adult Primary Care. *Prim Care Companion J Clin Psychiatry.* 2003;5:153-157.

78. Zuvekas SH. Prescription drugs and the changing patterns of treatment for mental disorders, 1996-2001. *Health Aff (Millwood).* 2005;24:195-205.

79. Corey-Lisle PK, Nash R, Stang P, Swindle R. Response, partial response, and nonresponse in primary care treatment of depression. *Arch Intern Med.* 2004;164:1197-1204.

80. Thase ME, Entsuah AR, Rudolph RL. Remission rates during treatment with venlafaxine or selective serotonin reuptake inhibitors. *Br J Psychiatry.* 2001;178:234-241.

81. Thase ME, Haight BR, Richard N et al. Remission rates following antidepressant therapy with bupropion or selective serotonin reuptake inhibitors: a meta-analysis of original data from 7 randomized controlled trials. *J Clin Psychiatry.* 2005;66:974-981.

82. Casacalenda N, Perry JC, Looper K. Remission in major depressive disorder: a comparison of pharmacotherapy, psychotherapy, and control conditions. *Am J Psychiatry.* 2002;159(8):1354-1360.

83. Churchill R, Hunot V, Corney R et al. A systematic review of controlled trials of the effectiveness and cost-effectiveness of brief psychological treatments for depression. *Health Technol Assess.* 2001;5(35):1-173.

84. U.S.Department of Health and Human Services. Mental Health and Mental Health Disorder. 2nd ed ed. Washington, D.C.: U.S. Governement Priting Office; 2000.

85. Robinson WD, Geske JA, Prest LA, Barnacle R. Depression treatment in primary care. *J Am Board Fam Pract.* 2005;18:79-86.

86. Dobscha SK, Gerrity MS, Corson K, Bahr A, Cuilwik NM. Measuring adherence to depression treatment guidelines in a VA primary care clinic. *General Hospital Psychiatry* 2003 Aug; 25(4):230-7.

87. Simon GE. Evidence review: efficacy and effectiveness of antidepressant treatment in primary care. *Gen Hosp Psychiatry.* 2002;24:213-224.

88. Olfson M, Marcus SC, Tedeschi M, Wan GJ. Continuity of antidepressant treatment for adults with depression in the United States. *Am J Psychiatry.* 2006;163:101-108.

89. Solberg LI, Trangle MA, Wineman AP. Follow-up and follow-through of depressed patients in primary care: the critical missing components of quality care. *J Am Board Fam Pract.* 2005;18:520-527.

90. Anderson IM. Selective serotonin reuptake inhibitors versus tricyclic antidepressants: a meta-analysis of efficacy and tolerability. *J Affect Disord.* 2000;58(1):19-36.

91. Beasley CM, Jr., Nilsson ME, Koke SC, Gonzales JS. Efficacy, adverse events, and treatment discontinuations in fluoxetine clinical studies of major depression: a meta-analysis of the 20-mg/day dose. *J Clin Psychiatry.* 2000;61:722-728.

92. Gartlehner, G., Hansen, RN., Thieda, P, DeVeaugh-Geiss, A., Gaynes, BN, Krebs, EE, Morgan, LC, Lux, LJ, Shumate, JA, Monroe, LG, and Lohr, KN. Comparative Effectiveness of Second-generation Antidepressants in the Pharmacologic Treatment of Adult Depression. 7. 2007. Rockville, MD, Agency for Healthcare Research and Quality.

93. MacGillivray S, Arroll B, Hatcher S et al. Efficacy and tolerability of selective serotonin reuptake inhibitors compared with tricyclic antidepressants in depression treated in primary care: systematic review and meta-analysis. *BMJ.* 2003;326:1014.

94. Mottram P, Wilson K, Strobl J. Antidepressants for depressed elderly. *Cochrane Database of Systematic Reviews (1).* 2006.

95. Mulrow CD, Williams JW, Chiquette E et al. Efficacy of newer medications for treating depression in primary care patients. *Am J Med.* 2000;108(1):54-64.

96. Kroenke K, West SL, Swindle R et al. Similar effectiveness of paroxetine, fluoxetine, and sertraline in primary care: a randomized trial. *JAMA.* 2001;286:2947-2955.

97. Depression Guideline Panel. *Depression in Primary Care: Volume 2. Treatment of Major Depression.* AHCPR Publication No. 93-0550 ed. United States Department of Health and Human Services; Public Health Service; Agency for Health Care Policy and Research; 1993.

98. The Management of Major Depressive Disorder Working Group. Veterans Health Administration/Department of Defense Performance Measures for the Management of Major Depressive Disorder in Adults. 2000. Washington, Veterans Health Administration and the Department of Defense.

99. Work Group On Major Depressive Disorder. *Practice Guideline for the Treatment of Patients With Major Depressive Disorder, Second Edition.* second ed. Washington: American Psychiatric Publishing, Inc.; 2000.

100. Gilbody S, House AO, Sheldon TA. Screening and case finding instruments for depression. *Cochrane Database of Systematic Reviews (4).* 2005.

101. Gilbody S, Whitty P, Grimshaw J, Thomas R. Educational and organisational interventions to improve the management of depression in primary care. *JAMA.* 2003;289(23):3145-3151.

102. Coyne J, Palmer S, Sullivan P. Screening for Depression in Adults. *Ann Intern Med.* 2003;138:767-768.

103. Hickie IB, Davenport TA, Ricci CS. Screening for depression in general practice and related medical settings. *Med J Aust.* 2002;177 Suppl:S111-S116.

104. Harris RP, Helfand M, Woolf SH et al. Current methods of the US Preventive Services Task Force: a review of the process. *Am J Prev Med.* 2001;20:21-35.

105. Medicines and Healthcare Products Regulatory Agency. Report of the CSM Expert Working Group on the Safety of Selective Serotonin Reuptake Inhibitor Antidepressants. MHRA . 2004.

106. National Institute for Clinical Excellence. Guideline Development Methods: Information for National Collaborating Centres and Guideline Developers. 2004. London.

107. Oxman AD, Guyatt GH. Validation of an index of the quality of review articles. *J Clin Epidemiol.* 1991;44:1271-1278.

108. Pignone M, Gaynes B, Lohr K, Rushton JL, Mulrow C. Screening for Depression in Adults. *Ann Intern Med.* 2003;138:767-768.

109. Rost K. Improving depression outcomes in community primary care practice: A randomized trial of the QuEST intervention. *J Gen Intern Med.* 2001;16:143-149.

110. Wells KB, Sherbourne C, Schoenbaum M et al. Impact of disseminating quality improvement programs for depression in managed primary care: a randomized controlled trial. *JAMA 283(2):212-20.* 2000.

111. Whooley MA, Stone B. Randomized trial of case-finding for depression in elderly primary care patients. *Journal of general internal medicine : official journal of the Society for Research and Education in Primary Care Internal Medicine.* 2000;15:293-300.

112. Callahan CM, Hendrie HC, Dittus RS, Brater DC, Hui SL, Tierney WM. Improving treatment of late life depression in primary care: a randomized clinical trial. *J Am Geriatr Soc.* 1994;42:839-846.

113. Bergus GR, Hartz AJ, Noyes R, Jr. et al. The limited effect of screening for depressive symptoms with the PHQ-9 in rural family practices. *Journal of Rural Health* 2005. *21(4):303-9.*

114. Jarjoura D, Polen A, Baum E, Kropp D, Hetrick S, Rutecki G. Effectiveness of screening and treatment for depression in ambulatory indigent patients. *Journal of General Internal Medicine.* 2004;78-84.

115. Bosmans, Judith, de Bruijne, Martine, van Hout, Hein, van Marwijk, Harm, Beekman, Aartjan, Bouter, Lex, Stalman, Wim, and van Tulder, Maurits. Cost-Effectiveness of a Disease Management Program for Major Depression in Elderly Primary Care Patients. Journal of General Internal Medicine 2006; 21[10], 1020-1026.

116. Rubenstein LZ, Alessi CA, Josephson KR, Trinidad HM, Harker JO, Pietruszka FM. A randomized trial of a screening, case finding, and referral system for older veterans in primary care. *J Am Geriatr Soc.* 2007;55:166-174.

117. van Marwijk, H., grundmeijer hglm, and breuren MM. Guidelines on Depression of the Dutch College of General Practitioners. huisarts wet , 482-490. 1994.

118. Wells K, Sherbourne C, Schoenbaum M et al. Five-year impact of quality improvement for depression: Results of a group-level randomized controlled trial. *Arch Gen Psychiatry.* 2004;61:378-386.

119. Rost, K. Treatment effect. 2006.

120. Pinquart M, Duberstein PR, Lyness JM. Treatments for later-life depressive conditions: a meta-analytic comparison of pharmacotherapy and psychotherapy. *Am J Psychiatry.* 2006;163:1493-1501.

121. Wilson K, Mottram P, Sivanranthan A, Nightingale A. Antidepressant versus placebo for depressed elderly. *Cochrane Database Syst Rev.* 2000.

122. Cuijpers, Pim, van Straten, Annemieke, and Smit, Filip. Psychological treatment of late-life depression: A meta-analysis of randomized controlled trials. International Journal of Geriatric Psychiatry 2006; 21[12], 1139-1149.

123. Pinquart M, Sorensen S. How effective are psychotherapeutic and other psychosocial interventions with older adults? A meta-analysis. *Journal of Mental Health and Aging.* 2001;7:207-243.

124. Stone, M. and Jones, M. L. Clinical Review: Relationship Between Antidepressant Drugs and Suicidality in Adults. 2006.

125. Levenson, M and Holland, C. Statistical Evaluation of Suicidality in Adults Treated with Antidepressants. 2006.

126. Khan A, Khan S, Kolts R, Brown WA. Suicide rates in clinical trials of SSRIs, other antidepressants, and placebo: analysis of FDA reports. *Am J Psychiatry.* 2003;160:790-792.

127. Jick SS, Dean AD, Jick H. Antidepressants and suicide. *BMJ.* 1995;310:215-218.

128. Martinez C, Rietbrock S, Wise L et al. Antidepressant treatment and the risk of fatal and non-fatal self harm in first episode depression: nested case-control study. *BMJ.* 2005;330:389.

129. Simon GE, Savarino J, Operskalski B, Wang PS. Suicide risk during antidepressant treatment. *American Journal of Psychiatry 163(1):41-7.* 2006.

130. Fergusson D, Doucette S, Glass KC et al. Association between suicide attempts and selective serotonin reuptake inhibitors: systematic review of randomised controlled trials. *BMJ* 2005 *330(7488):396.*

131. GlaxoSmithKline. Paroxetine Adult Suicidality Analysis: Major Depressive Disorder and Non-Major Depressive Disorder. 2006.

132. Dalton SO, Sorensen HT, Johansen C. SSRIs and upper gastrointestinal bleeding: what is known and how should it influence prescribing? *CNS Drugs.* 2006;20:143-151.

133. de Abajo FJ, Rodriguez LA, Montero D. Association between selective serotonin reuptake inhibitors and upper gastrointestinal bleeding: population based case-control study. *BMJ.* 1999;319:1106-1109.

134. van Walraven C, Mamdani MM, Wells PS, Williams JI. Inhibition of serotonin reuptake by antidepressants and upper gastrointestinal bleeding in elderly patients: retrospective cohort study. *BMJ.* 2001;323:655-658.

135. Dalton SO, Johansen C, Mellemkjaer L, Norgard B, Sorensen HT, Olsen JH. Use of selective serotonin reuptake inhibitors and risk of upper gastrointestinal tract bleeding: a population-based cohort study. *Arch Intern Med.* 2003;163:59-64.

136. Tata LJ, Fortun PJ, Hubbard RB et al. Does concurrent prescription of selective serotonin reuptake inhibitors and non-steroidal anti-inflammatory drugs substantially increase the risk of upper gastrointestinal bleeding? *Aliment Pharmacol Ther.* 2005;22:175-181.

137. Hammad TA, Laughren TP, Racoosin JA. Suicide rates in short-term randomized controlled trials of newer antidepressants. *J Clin Psychopharmacol.* 2006;26:203-207.

138. Gunnell D, Saperia J, Ashby D. Selective serotonin reuptake inhibitors (SSRIs) and suicide in adults: meta-analysis of drug company data from placebo controlled, randomised controlled trials submitted to the MHRA's safety review. *BMJ.* 2005;330:385.

139. Saperia J, Ashby D, Gunnell D. Suicidal behaviour and SSRIs: updated meta-analysis. *BMJ.* 2006;332:1453.

140. Storosum JG, van Zwieten BJ, van den BW, Gersons BP, Broekmans AW. Suicide risk in placebo-controlled studies of major depression. *Am J Psychiatry.* 2001;158:1271-1275.

141. Melander H, Ahlqvist-Rastad J, Meijer G, Beermann B. Evidence b(i)ased medicine--selective reporting from studies sponsored by pharmaceutical industry: review of studies in new drug applications. *BMJ.* 2003;326:1171-1173.

142. Lexchin J, Bero LA, Djulbegovic B, Clark O. Pharmaceutical industry sponsorship and research outcome and quality: systematic review. *BMJ.* 2003;326:1167-1170.

143. Mackay FJ, Dunn NR, Mann RD. Antidepressants and the serotonin syndrome in general practice. *Br J Gen Pract.* 1999;49:871-874.

144. Sondergard L, Kvist K, Andersen PK, Kessing LV. Do antidepressants prevent suicide? *Int Clin Psychopharmacol.* 2006;21:211-218.

145. Mackay FJ, Dunn NR, Wilton LV, Pearce GL, Freemantle SN, Mann RD. A comparison of fluvoxamine, fluoxetine, sertraline and paroxetine examined by observational cohort studies. *Pharmacoepidemiol Drug Saf.* 1997;6:235-246.

146. Gibbons RD, Brown CH, Hur K, Marcus SM, Bhaumik DK, Mann JJ. Relationship between antidepressants and suicide attempts: an analysis of the Veterans Health Administration data sets.[see comment]. *Am J Psychiatry.* 2007;164:1044-1049.

147. Mackay FR, Dunn NR, Martin RM, Pearce GL, Freemantle SN, Mann RD. Newer antidepressants: a comparison of tolerability in general practice. *Br J Gen Pract.* 1999;49:892-896.

148. Jick H, Kaye JA, Jick SS. Antidepressants and the risk of suicidal behaviors. *JAMA.* 2004;292:338-343.

149. Csizmadi I, Collet J, Boivin J. Bias and Confounding in Pharmacoepidemiology. In: Strom B, ed. *Pharmacoepidemiology.* Fourth ed. Philadelphia: John Wiley & Sons, Ltd; 2005:791-809.

150. Didham RC, McConnell DW, Blair HJ, Reith DM. Suicide and self-harm following prescription of SSRIs and other antidepressants: confounding by indication. *Br J Clin Pharmacol.* 2005;60:519-525.

151. Medicines and Healthcare Products Regulatory Agency. Venlafaxine (Effexor) Summary of Basis for Regulatory Position. Medicines and Healthcare Products Regulatory Agency . 2006. 1-29-2007.

152. Solomon DA, Keller MB, Leon AC et al. Recovery from major depression. A 10-year prospective follow-up across multiple episodes. *Arch Gen Psychiatry.* 1997;54:1001-1006.

153. Layton D, Clark DW, Pearce GL, Shakir SA. Is there an association between selective serotonin reuptake inhibitors and risk of abnormal bleeding? Results from a cohort study based on prescription event monitoring in England. *Eur J Clin Pharmacol.* 2001;57:167-176.

154. Meijer WE, Heerdink ER, Nolen WA, Herings RM, Leufkens HG, Egberts AC. Association of risk of abnormal bleeding with degree of serotonin reuptake inhibition by antidepressants. *Arch Intern Med.* 2004;164:2367-2370.

155. Richards JB, Papaioannou A, Adachi JD et al. Effect of selective serotonin reuptake inhibitors on the risk of fracture. *Archives of Internal Medicine 2007; 167 (2):188 -94 .*

156. Gilbody S, Sheldon T, Wessely S. Should we screen for depression? *BMJ.* 2006;332:1027-1030.

157. Palmer SC, Coyne JC. Screening for depression in medical care: pitfalls, alternatives, and revised priorities. *J Psychosom Res.* 2003;54:279-287.

158. Schwenk TL, Coyne JC, Fechner-Bates S. Differences between detected and undetected patients in primary care and depressed psychiatric patients. *Gen Hosp Psychiatry.* 1996;18:407-415.

159. Oxman TE, Sengupta A. Treatment of minor depression. *Am J Geriatr Psychiatry.* 2002;10(3):256-264.

160. Swindle RW, Rao JK, Helmy A et al. Integrating clinical nurse specialists into the treatment of primary care patients with depression. [References]. *Int J Psychiatry Med.* 2003;33:17-37.

161. Rost K, Nutting P, Smith J, Coyne JC, Cooper-Patrick L, Rubenstein L. The role of competing demands in the treatment provided primary care patients with major depression. *Arch Fam Med.* 2000;9:150-154.

162. Kessler D, Lloyd K, Lewis G, Gray DP. Cross sectional study of symptom attribution and recognition of depression and anxiety in primary care. *BMJ.* 1999;318:436-439.

163. Meredith LS, Orlando M, Humphrey N, Camp P, Sherbourne CD. Are better ratings of the patient-provider relationship associated with higher quality care for depression? *Medical Care* 2001; *39(4):349-60.*

164. Simon GE, Fleck M, Lucas R, Bushnell DM. Prevalence and predictors of depression treatment in an international primary care study. *Am J Psychiatry.* 2004;161:1626-1634.

165. Williams JB, Spitzer RL, Linzer M et al. Gender differences in depression in primary care. *Am J Obstet Gynecol.* 1995;173:654-659.

166. Badamgarav E, Weingarten SR, Henning JM et al. Effectiveness of disease management programs in depression: a systematic review. *American Journal of Psychiatry* 2003; *160(12):2080 -90.*

167. Gensichen J, Beyer M, Muth C, Gerlach FM, Von KM, Ormel J. Case management to improve major depression in primary health care: a systematic review. *Psychol Med.* 2006;36:7-14.

168. Neumeyer-Gromen A, Lampert T, Stark K, Kallischnigg G. Disease management programs for depression: a systematic review and meta-analysis of randomized controlled trials. *Med Care.* 2004;42(12):1211 223-1221.

169. Williams JW, Jr., Gerrity M, Holsinger T, Dobscha S, Gaynes B, Dietrich A. Systematic review of multifaceted interventions to improve depression care. *Gen Hosp Psychiatry.* 2007;29:91-116.

170. Wang PS, Simon G, Kessler RC. The economic burden of depression and the cost-effectiveness of treatment. *Int J Methods Psychiatr Res.* 2003;12:22-33.

171. Solberg LI, Trangle MA, Wineman AP. Follow-up and follow-through of depressed patients in primary care: the critical missing components of quality care. *J Am Board Fam Pract.* 2005;18:520-527.

172. Unutzer J, Schoenbaum M, Druss BG, Katon WJ. Transforming mental health care at the interface with general medicine: report for the presidents commission. *Psychiatr Serv.* 2006;57:37-47.

173. Von Korff M, Goldberg D. Improving outcomes in depression. *BMJ.* 2001;323:948-949.

174. Rost K, Pyne JM, Dickinson LM, LoSasso AT. Cost-Effectiveness of Enhancing Primary Care Depression Management on an Ongoing Basis. *Annals of Family Medicine.* 2005;3:7-14.

175. Skultety KM, Zeiss A. The treatment of depression in older adults in the primary care setting: an evidence-based review. *Health Psychol.* 2006;25:665-674.

176. Hunkeler EM, Katon W, Tang L et al. Long term outcomes from the IMPACT randomised trial for depressed elderly patients in primary care. *BMJ.* 2006;332:259-263.

177. Alexopoulos GS, Katz IR, Bruce ML et al. Remission in depressed geriatric primary care patients: a report from the PROSPECT study. *American Journal of Psychiatry* 2005; *162(4):718-24.*

178. Katon WJ, Schoenbaum M, Fan MY et al. Cost-effectiveness of improving primary care treatment of late-life depression. *Arch Gen Psychiatry.* 2005;62:1313-1320.

179. Katon WJ, Unutzer J, Simon G. Treatment of depression in primary care: where we are, where we can go. *Med Care.* 2004;42:1153-1157.

180. Ernst CL, Goldberg JF. Antisuicide properties of psychotropic drugs: a critical review. *Harv Rev Psychiatry.* 2004;12:14-41.

181. Juurlink DN, Mamdani MM, Kopp A, Redelmeier DA. The risk of suicide with selective serotonin reuptake inhibitors in the elderly. *Am J Psychiatry.* 2006;163:813-821.

182. Barak Y, Olmer A, Aizenberg D. Antidepressants reduce the risk of suicide among elderly depressed patients. *Neuropsychopharmacology.* 2006;31:178-181.

183. Bruce ML, Ten Have TR, Reynolds CFI et al. Reducing Suicidal Ideation and Depressive Symptoms in Depressed Older Primary Care Patients: A Randomized Controlled Trial. *JAMA: Journal of the American Medical Association.* 2004;291:1081-1091.

184. Gaynes BN, West SL, Ford CA, Frame P, Klein J, Lohr KN. Screening for suicide risk in adults: a summary of the evidence for the U.S. Preventive Services Task Force. *Ann Intern Med.* 2004;140:822-835.

185. Schulberg HC, Lee PW, Bruce ML et al. Suicidal ideation and risk levels among primary care patients with uncomplicated depression. *Ann Fam Med.* 2005;3:523-528.

186. Milane MS, Suchard MA, Wong ML, Licinio J. Modeling of the temporal patterns of fluoxetine prescriptions and suicide rates in the United States. *PLoS Medicine / Public Library of Science.* 2006;3:e190.

187. Roy-Byrne PP, Perera P, Pitts CD, Christi JA. Paroxetine response and tolerability among ethnic minority patients with mood or anxiety disorders: a pooled analysis. *J Clin Psychiatry.* 2005;66:1228-1233.

188. Shi L, Thiebaud P, McCombs JS. The impact of unrecognized bipolar disorders for patients treated for depression with antidepressants in the fee-for-services California Medicaid (Medi-Cal) program. *J Affect Disord.* 2004;82:373-383.

189. Sherbourne CD, Wells KB, Duan N et al. Long-term effectiveness of disseminating quality improvement for depression in primary care. *Arch Gen Psychiatry.* 2001;58:696-703.

190. Rost K, Nutting PA, Smith J, Werner JJ. Designing and implementing a primary care intervention trial to improve the quality and outcome of care for major depression. *General Hospital Psychiatry* 2000 Apr; *22(2):66-77.*

191. Rost K, Nutting P, Smith JL, Elliott CE, Dickinson M. Managing depression as a chronic disease: a randomised trial of ongoing treatment in primary care. *BMJ.* 2002;325:934.

192. Beasley CM, Jr., Koke SC, Nilsson ME, Gonzales JS. Adverse events and treatment discontinuations in clinical trials of fluoxetine in major depressive disorder: an updated meta-analysis. *Clin Ther.* 2000;22:1319-1330.

193. Gilbody SM, Whitty PM, Grimshaw JM, Thomas RE. Improving the detection and management of depression in primary care. [Review] [103 refs]. *Quality & Safety in Health Care* 2003; *12(2):149-55.*

194. Oslin DW, Sayers S, Ross J et al. Disease management for depression and at-risk drinking via telephone in an older population of veterans. *Psychosomatic Medicine* 2003 Dec; *65(6):931-7.*

195. Datto CJ, Thompson R, Horowitz D, Disbot M, Oslin DW. The pilot study of a telephone disease management program for depression. *Gen Hosp Psychiatry.* 2003;25:169-177.

196. Katon WJ, Von Korff M, Lin EH et al. The Pathways Study: a randomized trial of collaborative care in patients with diabetes and depression. *Arch Gen Psychiatry.* 2004;61:1042-1049.

197. Fortney JC, Pyne JM, Edlund MJ et al. A randomized trial of telemedicine-based collaborative care for depression. *Journal of general internal medicine : official journal of the Society for Research and Education in Primary Care Internal Medicine.* 2007;22:1086-1093.

198. Wang PS, Simon GE, Avorn J et al. Telephone screening, outreach, and care management for depressed workers and impact on clinical and work productivity outcomes: a randomized controlled trial. *JAMA.* 2007;298:1401-1411.

199. Unutzer J, Katon W, Callahan CM et al. Collaborative care management of late-life depression in the primary care setting: a randomized controlled trial. *JAMA.* 2002;288:2836-2845.

200. Dietrich AJ, Oxman TE, Williams JW, Jr. et al. Going to scale: re-engineering systems for primary care treatment of depression. *Ann Fam Med.* 2004;2:301-304.

201. Hedrick SC, Chaney EF, Felker B et al. Effectiveness of collaborative care depression treatment in Veterans' Affairs primary care. *Journal of General Internal Medicine* 2003; *18(1):9-16.*

202. Katzelnick DJ, Simon GE, Pearson SD et al. Randomized trial of a depression management program in high utilizers of medical care. *Archives of Family Medicine.* 2000.

203. Hunkeler EM, Meresman JF, Hargreaves WA et al. Efficacy of nurse telehealth care and peer support in augmenting treatment of depression in primary care. *Archives of Family Medicine* 2000; *9(8):700-8.*

204. Simon GE, VonKorff M, Rutter C, Wagner E. Randomised trial of monitoring, feedback, and management of care by telephone to improve treatment of depression in primary care.[see comment]. *BMJ.* 2000;320:550-554.

205. Peveler R, George C, Kinmonth AL, Campbell M, Thompson C. Effect of antidepressant drug counselling and information leaflets on adherence to drug treatment in primary care: randomised controlled trial. *BMJ.* 1999;319:612-615.

206. Banerjee S, Shamash K, MacDonald AJ, Mann AH. Randomised controlled trial of effect of intervention by psychogeriatric team on depression in frail elderly people at home.[see comment]. *BMJ.* 1996;313:1058-1061.

207. Schulberg HC, Block MR, Madonia MJ et al. Treating major depression in primary care practice. Eight-month clinical outcomes. *Arch Gen Psychiatry.* 1996;53:913-919.

208. Katon W, Von KM, Lin E et al. Collaborative management to achieve treatment guidelines. Impact on depression in primary care. *JAMA.* 1995;273:1026-1031.

209. Katon W, Robinson P, Von KM et al. A multifaceted intervention to improve treatment of depression in primary care. *Arch Gen Psychiatry.* 1996;53:924-932.

210. Katon W, Von Korff M, Lin E et al. Stepped collaborative care for primary care patients with persistent symptoms of depression: a randomized trial. *Arch Gen Psychiatry.* 1999;56:1109-1115.

211. Blanchard MR WA. The effect of primary care nurse intervention upon older people screened as depressed. *International Journal of Geriatric Psychiatry* 1995; *10(4):289-298.*

212. Ell K, Unutzer J, Aranda M, Gibbs NE, Lee PJ, Xie B. Managing depression in home health care: a randomized clinical trial. *Home Health Care Serv Q.* 2007;26:81-104.

213. Finley PR, Rens HR, Pont JT et al. Impact of a collaborative care model on depression in a primary care setting: a randomized controlled trial. *Pharmacotherapy.* 2003;23:1175-1185.

214. Capoccia KL BDBDEACDSNKWSS. Randomized trial of pharmacist interventions to improve depression care and outcomes in primary care. *American journal of health-system pharmacy : AJHP : official journal of the American Society of Health-System Pharmacists.* 2004;364-372.

215. Adler DA, Bungay KM, Wilson IB et al. The impact of a pharmacist intervention on 6-month outcomes in depressed primary care patients. *General Hospital Psychiatry* 2004 Jun; *26(3):199-209.*

216. Dobscha SK, Corson K, Hickam DH, Perrin NA, Kraemer DF, Gerrity MS. Depression decision support in primary care: a cluster randomized trial. *Ann Intern Med*. 2006;145:477-487.

217. Brook OH, van HH, Stalman W et al. A pharmacy-based coaching program to improve adherence to antidepressant treatment among primary care patients. *Psychiatr Serv*. 2005;56:487-489.

218. Rollman BL, Hanusa BH, Lowe HJ, Gilbert T, Kapoor WN, Schulberg HC. A randomized trial using computerized decision support to improve treatment of major depression in primary care. *J Gen Intern Med*. 2002;17:493-503.

219. Haw C, Houston K, Townsend E, Hawton K. Deliberate self-harm patients with alcohol disorders: characteristics, treatment, and outcome. *Crisis: Journal of Crisis Intervention & Suicide* 2001 *22(3):93-101*.

220. Dowrick C. Does testing for depression influence diagnosis or management by general practitioners? *Fam Pract*. 1995;12:461-465.

221. Thompson C, Kinmonth AL, Stevens L et al. Effects of a clinical-practice guideline and practice-based education on detection and outcome of depression in primary care: Hampshire Depression Project randomised controlled trial.[see comment]. *Lancet* 2000; *355(9199):185-91*.

222. Brown JB, Shye D, McFarland BH, Nichols GA, Mullooly JP, Johnson RE. Controlled trials of CQI and academic detailing to implement a clinical practice guideline for depression. *Jt Comm J Qual Improv*. 2000;26:39-54.

223. Goldberg HI, Wagner EH, Fihn SD et al. A randomized controlled trial of CQI teams and academic detailing: can they alter compliance with guidelines? *Joint Commission Journal on Quality Improvement*. 1998 *24(3):130-42*.

224. Mann AH BR. An evaluation of practice nurses working with general practitioners to treat people with depression. *British Journal of General Practice*. 1998; *48(426):875-879*.

225. Coleman EA GLS. Chronic care clinics: a randomized controlled trial of a new model of primary care for frail older adults see comments. *Journal of the American Geriatrics Society*. 1999; *47(7):775*.

226. Bashir K, Blizard B, Bosanquet A, Bosanquet N, Mann A, Jenkins R. The evaluation of a mental health facilitator in general practice: effects on recognition, management, and outcome of mental illness. *Br J Gen Pract*. 2000;50:626-629.

227. Solberg LI, Fischer LR, Wei F et al. A CQI intervention to change the care of depression: a controlled study. *Eff Clin Pract*. 2001;4:239-249.

228. Arthur AJ, Jagger C, Lindesay J, Matthews RJ. Evaluating a mental health assessment for older people with depressive symptoms in general practice: a randomised controlled trial. *Br J Gen Pract*. 2002;52:202-207.

229. Desai MM, Rosenheck RA, Craig TJ. Case-finding for depression among medical outpatients in the Veterans Health Administration. *Med Care*. 2006;44:175-181.

230. Stagnitti, MN. Antidepressant Use in the U.S. Civilian Noninstitutionalized Population, 2002. Agency for Healthcare Research and Quality. Medical Expenditure Panel Survey, Statistical Brief #77. 1-7. 2005.

231. Stafford RS, MacDonald EA, Finkelstein SN. National Patterns of Medication Treatment for Depression, 1987 to 2001. *Prim Care Companion J Clin Psychiatry*. 2001;3:232-235.

232. Olfson M, Marcus SC, Druss B, Elinson L, Tanielian T, Pincus HA. National trends in the outpatient treatment of depression. *JAMA*. 2002;287:203-209.

233. Joo JH, Solano FX, Mulsant BH, Reynolds CF, Lenze EJ. Predictors of adequacy of depression management in the primary care setting. *Psychiatr Serv*. 2005;56:1524-1528.

234. Solberg LI, Fischer LR, Rush WA, Wei F. When depression is the diagnosis, what happens to patients and are they satisfied? *Am J Manag Care*. 2003;9:131-140.

235. The Cochrane Collaboration. The Cochrane Manual Issue 1, 2007. www.cochrance.org/admin/manual.htm . 11-15-2006. 12-28-2006.

236. Johnstone A, Goldberg D. Psychiatric screening in general practice. A controlled trial. *Lancet*. 1976;1:605-608.

237. Zung WW, Magill M, Moore JT, George DT. Recognition and treatment of depression in a family medicine practice. *J Clin Psychiatry*. 1983;44:3-6.

238. Lewis G, Sharp D, Bartholomew J, Pelosi AJ. Computerized assessment of common mental disorders in primary care: effect on clinical outcome. *Fam Pract*. 1996;13:120-126.

239. Reifler DR, Kessler HS, Bernhard EJ, Leon AC, Martin GJ. Impact of screening for mental health concerns on health service utilization and functional status in primary care patients. *Arch Intern Med*. 1996;156:2593-2599.

240. Rubenstein LV, Jackson-Triche M, Unutzer J et al. Evidence-based care for depression in managed primary care practices. *Health Aff (Millwood)*. 1999;18:89-105.

241. Simon GE, Katon WJ, Lin EH et al. Cost-effectiveness of systematic depression treatment among people with diabetes mellitus. *Archives of General Psychiatry* 2007; *64 (1):65 -72* .

# Detection and Treatment of Depression in Primary Care

**Summary.** Current mental health screening rates may be as high as 74 percent in primary care, according to Healthy People 2010 midcourse review.[84] Once a primary care provider has identified a patient as depressed almost 90% of providers recommend antidepressants, either alone or in combination with psychotherapy.[85,86] However, among those patients who initiate antidepressant use, 40-67 percent discontinue use within 3 months,[87-89] in real-world settings. This is considerably higher than discontinuation rates reported in the context of clinical trials, where early treatment discontinuations rates range from 16 to 29 percent.[46,72,75,90-96] Only 25 percent of patients receive follow-up visits meeting HEDIS criteria of 3 visits in the first 12 weeks.[87]

## Detailed Information.

*Current screening practices.* Although not specific to depression, Healthy People 2010 identified increased mental health screening in primary care as one of its mental health objectives. Midcourse review data published on their website (http://wonder.cdc.gov/data2010/) reported a baseline rate of 62 percent of adults being screened in 2000, with the goal of achieving a 68 percent screening rate by 2010. By 2003, they report a 74 percent rate of mental health screening. It is unclear what specific disorders are being screened for, but given the prevalence and burden of depression in primary care it seems likely that most general mental health screening programs would include probes for depression. The VA currently requires annual depression screening of patients who are not being treated for depression. A 2006 study of screening in a VA system[229] found that 85 percent of eligible patients were screened for depression during the past year.

*Current antidepressant use.* A household survey found that 57 percent of community dwelling depressed adults seek treatment for depression, and about half of these receive care in a general medical setting.[21] Once a primary care patient is identified as depressed, the majority of providers recommend antidepressants, either alone (52 percent of depressed patients) or in combination with psychotherapy (36 percent).[85] In 2002, 13.2 percent of the US civilian, noninstitutionalized, elderly population and 10.3 percent of non-elderly adults used an antidepressant.[230] Use of antidepressants was much more likely in white non-Hispanics (10.6 percent) than in black non-Hispanics (4.0 percent) or Hispanics (3.6 percent) and in females (11.4 percent) than in males (5.4 percent).[230]

*Trends in antidepressant use.* Concomitant with trends showing that more patients are seeing physicians for depression,[77,231] and more primary care physicians in particular,[231] several trends are apparent in antidepressants use. Greater numbers of patients are being treated with antidepressants, both overall[77,88,231] and relative to other forms of outpatient treatment.[88] SSRI use has increased in particular.[231]

The estimated number of US physician visits by patients with depression in the National Disease and Therapeutic Index increased from 14.4 million visits in 1987 to 24.5 million visits in 2001.[231] According to the National Ambulatory Medical Care Survey (NAMCS), the yearly prevalence of depression diagnoses in primary care increased from two percent of visits in 1989 to 3.3 percent of visits in 2000.[77] Similarly, the rate of outpatient treatment for depression increased three-fold from 1987 to 1997 (from 0.73 to 2.33 per 100 persons in the Medical Expenditure Panel Survey (MEPS), p<0.001).[88] Over a similar time period, the proportion of visits to primary care physicians for depression, relative to specialty care physicians, increased from 50 percent in 1987 to 64 percent in 2001.[231] Regarding antidepressant use specifically, the odds of antidepressant prescriptions in visits with depression diagnosis increased from 1989-2000 (R = 1.07; CI: 1.04, 1.10)[77] and the rate of antidepressant medication use in patients seeing a physician for depression increased from 70 to 89 percent[231] from 1987 to 2001. Similarly, in 1997 twice as many patients (from 37.3 to 74.5 percent, p<0.001) receiving outpatient care for depression received antidepressant medications than in 1987. Significantly fewer (71.1 to 60.2 percent, p=0.006) received psychotherapy, however, and there was also a reduction in outpatient visits (12.6 to 8.7 visits per year, p=0.05).[88,232]

Finally, a strong trend away from tricyclic antidepressants (TCAs) toward the use of selective serotonin reuptake inhibitors (SSRIs) and other newer agents is apparent. According to the National Disease and Therapeutic Index (NDTI), the proportion of TCAs prescribed for depression dropped from 47 percent in 1987 to 2.1 percent in 2001. At the same time, SSRI use rose from 9.7 percent in 1988 when they were introduced to 69 percent in 2001.[231]

*Adequacy of treatment.* Although a 2005 study of a primary care-based quality assurance program found that 71 to 75 percent of depression patients receiving antidepressants were maintained at adequate doses, and dosages were appropriately increased when depressive symptoms did not remit, this level of care may not be typical of most primary care in the US.[233] A naturalistic international study of depression care[164], for example, found in a setting determined to be "typical of local primary health care delivery" in Seattle, WA that only 38 percent of the patients who screened positive for depression and had their depression confirmed by a diagnostic interview and were not already being treated for depression received antidepressants, and only 49 percent received any treatment at all. Patients may also limit the benefits of treatment by stopping treatment early. A large-scale study using household interview data[88] found that 42.4 percent of patients discontinued their antidepressants within 30 days, and only a little over twenty five percent of patients continued taking their antidepressants for more than 90 days. Another review found that up to 50 percent patients who initiate antidepressant use discontinue taking them within 3 months.[87] In these cases, follow-up contact or case management may provide an important way to track patients for whom treatment isn't working.

Studies using followup contact as a treatment quality indicator, however, have found that followup contact with depressed patients in primary care settings is often lacking. A household survey[21] found that 27 percent of community dwelling adults who are depressed receive depression care in a general medical setting. Forty-one percent of depressed participants treated in primary care settings described care that the researchers rated as "minimally adequate." "Minimally adequate" was defined as either (1) at least four outpatient visits with any type of physician for pharmacotherapy that included use of either antidepressant or mood stabilizer for a minimum of 30 days, or (2) at least eight outpatient visits with any professional in the specialty mental health sector for psychotherapy lasting a mean of at least 30 minutes. No time-frame was specified for these visits. Sixty-four percent of the patients treated in specialty mental health settings received "minimally adequate" care.

A 2003 study[234] looked at usual depression care at a large staff-model medical group in Minnesota. Researchers surveyed patients who had been given a depression diagnosis at a visit during the past week about their depression care. Seventy-eight percent of the patients contacted reported that they were taking antidepressants at the time they completed the one-week post-visit questionnaire. At least 42 percent of the patients were taking antidepressants at the time of their index visit, according to chart audit, so most of these were not new prescriptions. At 3-month followup, 24 percent of the patients re-surveyed reported having received a new prescription for an antidepressant, and 67 percent of these reported that they stopped taking their antidepressants before a clinician told them to stop.[89] Regarding followup appointments, 59 percent of the patients had at least one followup visit during the subsequent 3 months, and 10 percent had three or more visits. Nearly all of those with three or more visits were seeing mental health therapists rather than primary care clinicians.[234] It is difficult to determine from these data the proportion likely to have received "minimally adequate" care according to the community survey definition, but it seems unlikely that it would exceed the 41 percent reported by the community survey study described above.

Another 2003 study looked at adherence to evidence-based guidelines in the VA system,[86] where annual depression screening of patients without known depression is the standard of care. They identified nineteen indicators of guideline-concordant care based on guidelines published by AHPCR,[17,97] Veteran's Health Administration (VA),[98] and the American Psychiatric Association (APA)[99] that could be documented in the medical chart, such as exploration of functional limitations or current social stressors, discussion of treatment preferences and options, phone or in-person contact with primary care staff within 2 weeks, and evaluation of depressive symptoms between 12 and 24 weeks. They found that approximately half of the items were completed on average, with some items being completed on only 13.5 percent of the sample (contact within two weeks) and some being completed for 100 percent of the sample (noting a positive screen or exploring depression; initiating or discussing treatment). Other indicators that were met a substantial (>65 percent) portion of the time include exploration of functional limitations or social stressors; assessing drug and alcohol use; completing a physical exam; lab-work of potential relevance to depressed mood; and initiating or offering treatment. Thus, the assessment process appears to be fairly thorough, although review of specific DSM-IV or PHQ symptoms was documented in only 46 percent of the charts.

Treatment discussion and/or initiation were documented in all cases, and 63 percent of patients were prescribed antidepressants, fewer than the 78 percent reporting antidepressant use in the Minnesota HMO study. Seventy-three percent of the VA patients filled at least 90 days of the medication and reached a therapeutic dosage, and the average number of mental health visits was 3.4, among the 40 percent who saw mental health providers. It is difficult to say how many of these patients would have met the criteria for "minimally adequate" care as defined by the community survey, but it may be consistent with the 41 percent seen in the community survey.

In this sample they also collected followup Patient Health Questionnaire (PHQ), data on 46 percent of the patients, an average of 8.6 months after the initial PHQ. Only two of the 51 completing the followup questionnaire met criteria for remission at followup, though this number must be interpreted with caution given the low followup rate.

**Appendix B. USPSTF Hierarchy of research design and quality rating criteria.**[104]

**Hierarchy of Research Design**

| | |
|---|---|
| I | Properly conducted randomized controlled trial (RCT) |
| II-1: | Well-designed controlled trial without randomization |
| II-2: | Well-designed cohort or case-control analytic study |
| II-3: | Multiple time series with or without the intervention; dramatic results from uncontrolled experiments |
| III: | Opinions of respected authorities, based on clinical experience; descriptive studies or case reports; reports of expert committees |

**Design-Specific Criteria**

**Systematic Reviews**

**Criteria:**
- Comprehensiveness of sources considered/search strategy used
- Standard appraisal of included studies
- Validity of conclusions
- Recency and relevance are especially important for systematic reviews

**Case-Control Studies**

**Criteria:**
- Accurate ascertainment of cases
- Nonbiased selection of cases/controls with exclusion criteria applied equally to both
- Response rate
- Diagnostic testing procedures applied equally to each group
- Measurement of exposure accurate and applied equally to each group
- Appropriate attention to potential confounding variables

**Randomized Controlled Trials and Cohort Studies**

**Criteria:**
- Initial assembly of comparable groups
  - -for RCTs: adequate randomization, including first concealment and whether potential confounders were distributed equally among groups.
  - -for cohort studies: consideration of potential confounders with either restriction or measurement for adjustment in the analysis; consideration of inception cohorts
- Maintenance of comparable groups (includes attrition, crossovers, adherence, contamination)
- Important differential loss to follow-up or overall high loss to follow-up
- Measurements: equal, reliable, and valid (includes masking of outcome assessment)
- Clear definition of the interventions
- All important outcomes considered

**Diagnostic Accuracy Studies**

**Criteria:**
- Screening test relevant, available for primary care, adequately described
- Study uses a credible reference standard, performed regardless of test results
- Reference standard interpreted independently of screening test
- Handles indeterminate result in a reasonable manner
- Spectrum of patients included in study
- Sample size
- Administration of reliable screening test

**Appendix B Table 1. Specific Quality Rating Criteria**

| Randomized Controlled Trials | Systematic Reviews |
|---|---|
| Random assignment | Is there a clear review question? |
| Allocation concealment | Was the literature search strategy stated |
| Groups similar at baseline | Were there explicit inclusion/exclusion criteria reported relating to selection of the primary studies |
| Eligibility criteria specified | Selection Bias |
| Clear definition of Intervention | Is there evidence of a substantial effort to search for all relevant research |
| Training of treatment providers reported | Is the validity of included studies adequately assessed |
| Supervision of treatment providers reported | Is sufficient detail of the individual studies presented |
| Patient and provider treatment allegiance or preference reported | Are any important studies missing |
| Blinded outcomes assessors | Are the primary studies summarized appropriately |
| Attrition <40% and not differential | Were the authors' conclusions supported by the evidence they presented |
| Adherence reported | What was the funding source and role of funder |
| Cross-over reported | |
| Likelihood of contamination | |
| Appropriate statistical analysis | |

**Appendix C. Inclusion and exclusion criteria for key questions.**

**Key Question 1 and 1a-Screening trials**
**Inclusion Criteria:**
1. Screening: study of depression screening; outcomes same as those listed above.

**Exclusion Criteria:**
1. Focus on inpatient, residential treatment, psychiatric, or community settings.
2. Focus on interventions that are not primary care feasible or referable (e.g. ECT).
3. Does not meet quality criteria, including follow-up of less than 6 weeks.
4. Focus on children or adolescents.
5. None of the outcomes listed above.
6. Focus on pregnancy-related screening.
7. Examination of genetic modifiers.
8. Does not meet any inclusion criterion.
9. Not a general primary care population.
10. Not English language or non-developed country.
11. Non-comparative study/excluded design.
12. Comparative-effectiveness study.
13. Missing both depression-specific screener and depression-specific outcome.
14. Use as source document.
15. Screen not used in clinical care.

**Key Question 2-Harms of screening**
**Inclusion Criteria:**
1. Study addressing <u>adverse events</u> associated with depression screening.

**Exclusion Criteria:**
1. Setting limits generalizability to general adult primary care population.
2. Focus on interventions other than antidepressants
3. Does not meet quality criteria, including follow-up of less than 6 weeks
4. Focus on children or adolescents.
5. Focus on pregnancy-related screening.
6. Examination of genetic modifiers.
7. Does not meet any inclusion criterion.
8. Not generalizable to primary care population
9. Not English language or non-developed country
10. Non-comparative study/excluded design.
11. Use as source document

**Key Question 3-Treatment with antidepressants in the elderly**
**Inclusion Criteria:** Study of <u>depression treatment</u> with antidepressants in the elderly, meeting **all** of the following criteria:
1. Setting: primary care, outpatient mental health, community setting if intervention is PC-feasible or referable.
2. Intervention: antidepressant for acute treatment of depression
3. Quality: fair-good quality per USPSTF standards, with follow-up of at least 6 weeks.
4. Design: Meta-analysis or systematic evidence review
5. Outcomes: depressive symptomatology, quality of life ratings, assessments of functioning, depressive illness diagnosis, suicidality (attempts or ideation), or change in health status (e.g., death, improvement in co-morbid disorders, reduction in physical complaints).
6. Population: Exclusively or primarily (> 80%) ages 65 and older
7. Context/Environment: Conducted in US, UK, Canada, Australia, New Zealand
8. Language: Published in English

**Exclusion Criteria:**
1. Focus on inpatient, residential treatment, psychiatric, or community settings.
2. Focus on interventions that are not primary-care feasible or referable
3. Does not meet quality criteria, including follow-up of less than 6 weeks
4. Focus on children or adolescents
5. None of the outcomes listed above.
6. Examination of genetic modifiers
7. Does not meet any inclusion criterion.
8. Not a general primary care population

9. Not English language or one of included countries
10. Non-comparative study.
11. Comparative-effectiveness study.
12. Use as source document
13. Focus on non-elderly adults.
14. Depression prevention or treatment maintenance interventions.
15. Not a treatment outcomes study.
16. Article is an individual trial (rather than synthesized review), or it is a SER/MA with content area covered more comprehensively or recently in one of the Included reviews.

## Key Question 3-Treatment with psychotherapy in the elderly

**Inclusion Criteria**: Study of <u>depression treatment</u> with psychotherapy in the elderly, meeting **all** of the following criteria:
1. Setting: primary care, outpatient mental health, community setting if intervention is PC-feasible or referable.
2. Intervention: cognitive-behavioral, interpersonal therapy, or problem-solving type intervention
3. Quality: fair-good quality per USPSTF standards, with follow-up of at least 6 weeks.
4. Design: Systematic evidence review or meta-analysis
5. Outcomes: depressive symptomatology, quality of life ratings, assessments of functioning, depressive illness diagnosis, suicidality (attempts or ideation), or change in health status (e.g., death, improvement in co-morbid disorders, reduction in physical complaints).
6. Population: Exclusively or primarily (> 80%) ages 65 and older
7. Context/Environment: Conducted in US, UK, Canada, Australia, New Zealand
8. Language: Published in English

**Exclusion Criteria, any of the following**:
1. Focus on inpatient, residential treatment, psychiatric, or community settings.
2. Focus on interventions that are not primary-care feasible or referable
3. Does not meet quality criteria, including follow-up of less than 6 weeks
4. Focus on children or adolescents
5. None of the outcomes listed above
6. Examination of genetic modifiers
7. Does not meet any inclusion criterion.
8. Not a general primary care population
9. Not English language or one of included countries
10. Non-comparative study.
11. Comparative-effectiveness study.
12. Use as source document
13. Focus on interventions that are not primarily CBT-related or IPT in nature (e.g., pharmacotherapy, reminiscence, psychodynamic)
14. Focus on non-elderly adults.
15. Depression prevention or treatment maintenance interventions.
16. Not a treatment outcomes study.
17. Article is an individual trial (rather than synthesized review), or it is a SER/MA with content area covered more comprehensively or recently in one of the Included reviews.

## Key Question 4-Harms of Depression Treatment with Antidepressants
**Inclusion Criteria**:
1. Systematic review, regulatory review, large cohort, or large prospective observational study addressing <u>adverse events</u> associated with depression treatment or screening.
2. For studies of suicidality:
   a. Minimum n=10,000 for cohort or observational study
   b. Minimum follow-up=6 months
3. For studies of non-suicidality harms
   a. Minimum n=1,000 for cohort or observational studies
   b. Minimum follow-up=3 months
   c. May include comparative effectiveness without control group if provides absolute rates of harms in an understudied population

**Exclusion Criteria**:
1. Focus on inpatient, residential treatment, psychiatric, or community settings.
2. Focus on interventions that are not primary care feasible or referable (e.g. ECT)

3. Does not meet quality criteria, including follow-up of less than 6 weeks
4. Focus on children or adolescents
5. None of the adverse effects of interest to our review above.
6. Focus on pregnancy-related screening.
7. Updated/covered by another more recent MA/SR
8. Does not meet any inclusion criterion.
9. Not a general primary care population
10. Not English language or non-developed country
11. Not a study design specified above.
12. Comparative-effectiveness study.
13. Use as source document
14. Use as a discussion document only.

# Key Questions and Analytic Framework

Using the USPSTF methods, we developed an analytic framework (Figure1) to guide our literature search. This review focused on five KQs related to this analytic framework that the USPSTF determined needed to be updated for its recommendation.

## Critical Key Questions Addressed in This Update

KQ1. Is there direct evidence that screening for depression among adults and the elderly in primary care reduces morbidity (including improved depression response and remission) and/or mortality?

KQ1a. What is the impact of clinician feedback of screening test results (with our without additional care management support) on depression response and remission in screen-detected depressed patients receiving primary care?

KQ2. What are the adverse effects of screening for depressive disorders in adults and the elderly?

KQ3. Is antidepressant and/or psychotherapy treatment of elderly depressed patients effective in improving health outcomes?

KQ4. What are the adverse effects of antidepressant treatment (suicidality, psychiatric hospitalization, and discontinuation of medication due to adverse events) for depression in adults and the elderly?

## Key Questions Not Updated in This Review

- Efficacy of treatment in adults
- Accuracy of screening instruments in adults and older patients

# Literature Search Strategy

We initially searched for systematic evidence reviews (SERs) and meta-analyses (MAs) on depression treatment or screening in adults and elderly in Pubmed-Medline from 1998 through December 2007 and in the Database of Abstracts of Reviews (DARE), and Cochrane Database of Systematic Review (CDSR) in October, 2005, with an updated search in October, 2006 to capture studies published in the interim. We screened systematic reviews (SR) and meta analyses (MA) at the abstract stage and at the article review stage for relevance to each of our key questions and for quality (Appendix C for inclusion/exclusion criteria).

Subsequent searches specific to each key question were done to supplement evidence found in the search of reviews and meta-analyses. All searches were examined by two reviewers for relevance to all key questions. We also hand-searched the Robert Wood Johnson Foundation and the MacArthur Foundation websites, as well as reviewing the National Institute for Health and Clinical Excellence guideline for management of depression in primary and secondary care and its complete bibliography.[57]

**Appendix D. Detailed methods.**

For KQ1 and KQ1a, none of the systematic reviews of depression screening were wholly consistent with our inclusion-exclusion parameters. We, therefore, conducted a primary literature search to cover the time period since the previous USPSTF review (1998 through December, 2007) for controlled trials (RCTs and CCTs) of depression screening in primary care settings in Ovid-Medline, Psychinfo, and Cochrane Collaboration Registry of Controlled Trials (CCRCT). Search terms are listed in Appendix D Table 1. In addition, in order to locate other screening trials for KQ1, comparing screened and a non-screened groups, we searched Ovid-Medline, Science Citation Index, Social Science Citation Index, Science Direct, HighWire Press, and Google Scholar from 2000 to March, 2006 for articles referencing the single screening article from the previous USPSTF review that included a non-screened control group.[10] We also evaluated all trials that involved screening and reported health outcomes in the previous USPSTF review[1,71] the 2005 Cochrane review on depression screening,[100] and a recent review on educational and organizational interventions for depression.[101]

For KQ2, we searched all abstracts found for KQ1 and KQ1a and all articles pulled for further examination for KQ1 and KQ1a for evidence of harms. We also examined systematic and non-systematic reviews for evidence of harms or potential harms. Additionally, we searched Ovid-Medline, PubMed, and Psychinfo from 1998 through December, 2007 using the same search terms as KQ1 and KQ1a except without restrictions on study design, and adding terms to capture harms generally (i.e., adverse events, harms), and one specific potential harm suggested in review articles (labeling).

For KQ3, in addition to the initial SER search described above, we searched Ovid-Medline, PsycINFO, and CCRCT specifically for controlled trials, systematic reviews, or meta-analyses of psychotherapy and antidepressant treatment in the elderly in two separate searches covering 1998- December, 2007 for psychotherapy trials and 2003-December, 2007 for antidepressant trials. (We only searched for original trials beginning in 2003 for antidepressant treatment because we found one meta-analysis in our original SER search that covered trials published through 2004.) Reference lists of all articles reviewed from these searches were hand-searched for potentially relevant trials or systematic reviews. We reviewed abstracts and articles from three meta-analyses that met our inclusion criteria and appeared to capture the relevant trials comprehensively. Because these meta-analyses were recent and comprehensive we used them as our evidence for this question rather than using individual trials.

For KQ4, in addition to the initial search for SERs and MAs and hand searches described above, we reviewed all abstracts located for KQ1, KQ2, and KQ3 for treatment-associated harms and used one comparative effectiveness review of second generation antidepressants[92] and one evidence-based depression care guideline[57] as source documents for systematic reviews and primary articles addressing harms. Additionally, we searched MEDLINE and PsycINFO from 1988 through December, 2007 to locate large (minimum of 10,000 observations and 6 months of followup for suicide-related harms, and minimum 1000 observations and 3 months of followup for non-suicide-related harms) observational studies addressing adverse effects by searching for publications that included SSRI terms and terms related to either suicide or discontinuation without restrictions related to study design.

# Inclusion/Exclusion Criteria

We developed a set of inclusion/exclusion criteria that were applied to each key questions, with specific criteria for inclusion and exclusion as needed for each key question.

**Appendix D. Detailed methods.**

*Populations and Disorders.* The population of interest: general population non-pregnant adults (ages 18 and over) treated in primary care setting in the US, Canada, UK, Australia, New Zealand, for non-synthesized literature, with inclusion of studies from other northern European countries when data were not adequate for a specific key question. Diagnostic categories of interest: Major Depressive Disorder, Dysthymia, and Depression Not Otherwise Specified (including Minor Depression), or "depression" with no further diagnostic specificity. We did not include studies with a primary focus on pregnancy-related depression, Bipolar Disorders, Schizoaffective disorder, Seasonal Affective Disorder, Cyclothymia, Substance-Induced Mood Disorder, or Adjustment Disorder with depressed mood. We excluded studies focusing only on patients at high-risk for depression and those focused exclusively on Dysthymia or Minor Depression.

*Settings.* Primary care or community practices. We excluded studies conducted exclusively in inpatient, residential treatment, psychiatric, or non-health care community settings (e.g. worksites).

*Screening (KQ1/1a, KQ2).* We included RCTs/CCTs of screening programs comparing screened vs. unscreened patients, and RCTs/CCTs in screened-detected patients examining the health outcomes from screening and feedback of test results to primary care clinicians, with or without other depression care supports. Screening studies were required to use a depression-specific screening instrument or, if no depression-specific screener is used then they must report depression-specific outcomes. We excluded any system-level, Q.I., or depression care management interventions that did not involve screening. Screening trials must have used the screening results in the care of the intervention participants and must not have used the screening results in the care of the control participants.

*Treatments (KQ3, KQ4).* To be consistent with the previous review for the USPSTF, we limited treatments to antidepressant medications, psychotherapy, or combinations of these two for KQ3. We limited medication treatments to antidepressants, excluding mood stabilizers such as lithium, valproic acid, and Carbamazepine. For harms (KQ4), we focused on antidepressants only, and on newer ("second-generation") antidepressant in particular.

*Outcomes.* For all key questions except KQ4, health outcomes of interest included: depressive symptomatology (response), quality of life ratings, assessments of functioning, change in fulfilling criteria for the diagnosis of a study-relevant depressive illness (remission), suicidality (attempts or ideation), or change in health status (e.g., death, improvement in co-morbid disorders, reduction in physical complaints). We did not consider recognition or treatment of depression as health outcomes. For KQ4, we focused on suicide-related events, serious psychiatric events, serious medical events (for older adults), and discontinuation (overall and due to adverse events).

*Study Designs.* For KQ1 and KQ1a we limited our searches to RCTs and well-designed, non-randomized controlled trials. Designs for key question 2 included RCTs, CCTs, and high-quality observational studies. Evidence for KQ3 was limited to high-quality recent meta-analyses. For KQ4, we included systematic reviews, regulatory reviews, or meta-analyses of RCTs and large observational studies (minimum of 10,000 observations and 6 months of followup for suicide-related harms, and minimum 1000 observations and 3 months of followup for non-suicide-related harms).

*Quality.* We excluded studies that met criteria for "Poor" quality using the USPSTF design-specific criteria.

*Language.* We excluded non-English language abstracts and articles.

*Costs.* We retrieved articles on cost and cost-effectiveness relevant to depression screening in primary care.


# Literature Review Process

We reviewed a total of 4088 abstracts and 412 complete articles for all KQs (Appendix D Figure 1). Abstracts were reviewed by two investigators against inclusion/exclusion criteria specific for each key question. Retrieved articles were compared to inclusion and exclusion criteria by two investigators for the applicable key question(s). Included studies that met all criteria were then rated by two raters for quality according to USPSTF standards.[104] Separate criteria were used to judge quality of original research articles and systematic reviews. The rating process involved the independent examination of several key quality indicators listed in Appendix B Table 1. Articles were rated as good (no notable flaws), fair (minor flaws) or poor, (major flaw(s) or numerous minor flaws) by each rater, and disagreements were settled by consensus.

For KQ1 and KQ1a we examined 248 articles, and of these retained one trial for KQ1 and seven trials for KQ1a. Five of the KQ1 and KQ1a studies were included in the 2002 USPSTF review, and three additional studies were found from our database searches. Hierarchical inclusion criteria for KQ1a are presented in Appendix D Figure 2. Briefly, we included trials that screened consecutively or randomly selected adult patients in a primary care setting. Screening instruments were required to be specific to depression or to include a module specific to depression. Studies ranged considerably in the extensiveness of the depression education and care supports provided in addition to screening and feedback. We included studies, regardless of the level of additional intervention, as long as screening results were used in the clinical care of the patient. We excluded studies that screened high-risk populations rather than general populations. An unscreened control group was required for KQ1, but for KQ1a the control group was screened but without results being systematically returned to the provider.

For KQ2 we included studies that measured adverse events related to depression screening. We did not find any studies in any of the searches used for KQ2 that met our inclusion-exclusion criteria for harms of screening.

For KQ3 we included controlled trials or systematic reviews of antidepressant or psychotherapy treatment in populations of older patients. We excluded studies that focused on specific high risk groups, such as stroke patients. We retained three systematic reviews that included meta-analyses.

For KQ4, we limited our review to systematic or regulatory reviews of RCTS reporting specific, serious harms (suicidality, psychiatric morbidity and, in the elderly, medical morbidity) and tolerability (early discontinuation overall and due to adverse effects) as a proxy for a large range of common, less serious adverse events. We supplemented synthesized short-term trial data with large observational studies.

For suicide-related adverse events, we included one systematic review and five regulatory reviews from our SER search, from our searches for other key questions, and from hand-searches. Two types of reviews were included: 1) regulatory reviews, which included all clinical trials submitted to national regulatory agencies by the manufacturers to support drug approval, with reviews conducted by the agency or by outside investigators; and 2) published systematic reviews, that may not include all unpublished regulatory trials, but may also include RCTs that are funded by an agency other than the drug's manufacturer.

For serious psychiatric events (e.g. hospitalization), we did not find any existing systematic reviews, but included one large clinical trial (STAR-D) and one uncontrolled trial.

For serious medical events in the elderly, we located one systematic review of upper gastrointestinal bleeding.

For tolerability, we located seven systematic reviews or meta-analyses and two cohort or uncontrolled trials which reported discontinuation (overall and due to adverse events).

## Data Abstraction

One primary reviewer abstracted relevant information into standardized evidence tables for each included article for KQ1 and KQ1a combined, KQ3, and KQ4 (in two tables: one for meta-analyses and one for cohort and observational studies) (Appendix G). A second reviewer checked the abstracted data for accuracy and completeness.

## Literature Synthesis

We did not conduct quantitative synthesis for any key question, although we relied extensively on these data from published meta-analyses for KQ3 (treatment in the elderly) and KQ4 (adverse effects of treatment). For KQ4, we abstracted data to calculate absolute event rates for suicide-related events were abstracted from meta-analyses and systematic reviews, with 95 percent CI calculated based on a Poisson distribution using the SAS version 8.2 GENMOD procedure with the offset option set at the log of the event rate. Risk differences with 95 percent CI for suicide-related events in patients with MDD (a relatively homogeneous risk group) on active medication were calculated using the RISKDIFF option of the FREQ procedure in SAS 8.2. This procedure uses a normal approximation to the binomial distribution to construct asymptotic confidence intervals (SAS Version 8.2 for Windows, SAS Institute Inc., Cary, North Carolina). The only key questions for which we relied solely on original research was KQ1 and KQ1a. For KQ1a, we did not attempt meta-analysis of results as we judged that the included studies displayed too much clinical diversity (e.g. screening instruments, extent of the interventions, and populations) and methodological diversity (e.g., comparability of intervention and control groups across studies) to be synthesized quantitatively (Appendix F).[235] Instead, we qualitatively synthesized our results, discussing studies with a focus on elderly patients separately.

**Appendix D Figure 1. Search results and article flow by key question.**

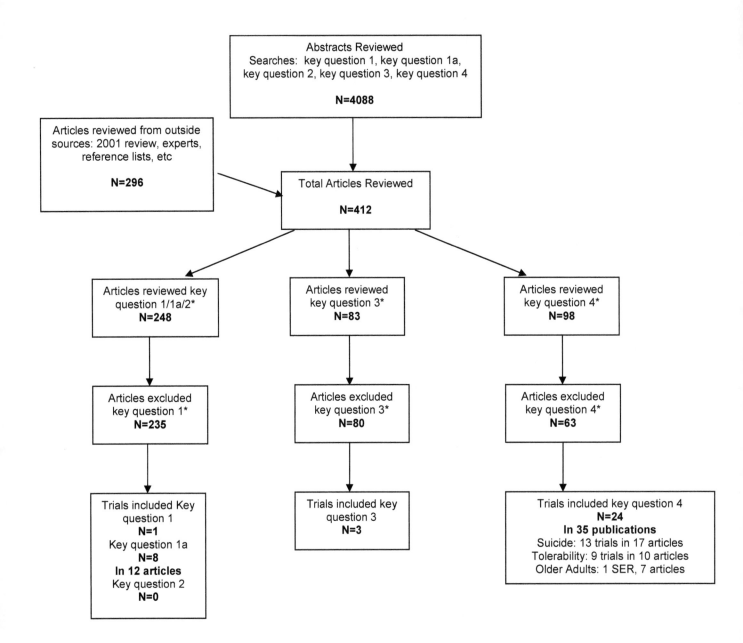

* Overlap occurs between the articles reviewed for each key question.

**Appendix D Table 1. Search Strategies.**

**Systematic Review**
Databases: MedLine, Cochrane Database of Systematic Reviews, Database of Abstracts of Reviews of Effects
Dates: 1998 to December 2007

1  depression/dt [drug therapy] OR depression/pc[prevention and control] OR depression/rh[rehabilitation] OR depression/th[therapy]

2  depression, postpartum/dt[drug therapy] OR depression, postpartum/pc[prevention and control] OR depression, postpartum/rh[rehabilitation] OR depression, postpartum/th[therapy]

3  depressive disorder, major/dt[drug therapy] OR depressive disorder, major/pc[prevention and control] OR depressive disorder, major/rh[rehabilitation] OR depressive disorder, major/th[therapy]

4  dysthymic disorder/dt[drug therapy] OR dysthymic disorder/pc[prevention and control] OR dysthymic disorder/rh[rehabilitation] OR dysthymic disorder/th[therapy]

5  depressive disorder/dt[drug therapy] OR depressive disorder/pc[prevention and control] OR depressive disorder/rh[rehabilitation] OR depressive disorder/th[therapy]

6  depression/ OR depressive disorder OR depression, postpartum/ OR depressive disorder, major/ OR dysthymic disorder/

7  "mass screening" OR screen$.ti,ab

8  6 AND 7

9  1 OR 2 OR 3 OR 4 OR 5 OR 8

10  9 AND systematic[sb] Field: All Fields, Limits: All Adult: 19+ years, Publication Date from 1998 to 2006, English

11  9 AND systematic[sb]


**Screening Trials**
Database: MedLine, PsychInfo, Cochrane Central Register of Controlled Trials
Dates: 1996 to December 2007

1  Depression/
2  Depressive Disorder/
3  Depressive Disorder, Major/
4  1 or 2 or 3
5  Mass Screening/
6  screen$.ti,ab.
7  case finding.ti,ab.
8  casefinding.ti,ab.
9  5 or 6 or 7 or 8
10  4 and 9
11  Mental Disorders/di
12  depress$.ti,ab.
13  9 and 11 and 12
14  10 or 13
15  limit 14 to (clinical trial or controlled clinical trial or randomized controlled trial)
16  clinical trials/ or controlled clinical trials/ or randomized controlled trials/
17  double-blind method/ or random allocation/ or single-blind method/
18  random$.ti,ab.
19  16 or 17 or 18
20  14 and 19
21  15 or 20
22  limit 21 to english language
23  limit 22 to yr="1998 - 2006"


**Screening Harms**
Database: Ovid MEDLINE(R), PubMed, PsychInfo
Dates: 1966 to December 2007

1  Depression/
2  Depressive Disorder/
3  Depressive Disorder, Major/
4  Mental Disorders/di [Diagnosis]
5  depress$.ti,ab.
6  4 and 5
7  1 or 2 or 3 or 6

8    Mass Screening/
9    screen$.ti,ab.
10   case finding.ti,ab.
11   casefinding.ti,ab.
12   8 or 9 or 10 or 11
13   7 and 12
14   adverse effects.fs.
15   adverse effect$.ti,ab.
16   harm$.ti,ab.
17   label$.ti,ab.
18   14 or 15 or 16 or 17
19   13 and 18
20   limit 19 to english language
21   limit 20 to yr="1998 - 2006"

**Elderly-Treatment trials**
Database: Ovid MEDLINE(R), PsycInfo, Cochrane Central Register of Controlled Trials
Dates: 1998- December 2007
1    Depression
2    Depressive Disorder, Major
3    Depressive Disorder
4    depress$.ti,ab
5    Mental Disorders
6    4 and 5
7    1 or 2 or 3 or 6
8    Psychotherapy/
9    Behavior Therapy/
10   Cognitive Therapy/
11   Psychotherapy, Brief/
12   Counseling/
13   Directive Counseling/
14   Problem Solving/
15   psychotherap$.ti,ab.
16   (behavi$ and (therap$ or treatment$ or intervention$)).ti,ab.
17   (Cognitive and (therap$ or treatment$ or intervention$)).ti,ab.
18   interpersonal therap$.ti,ab.
19   interpersonal psychotherap$.ti,ab.
20   interpersonal intervention$.ti,ab.
21   counsel$.ti,ab.
22   problem solving.ti,ab.
23   8 or 9 or 10 or 11 or 12 or 13 or 14 or 15 or 16 or 17 or 18 or 19 or 20 or 21 or 22
24   aged/ or "aged, 80 and over"/ or frail elderly/
25   older.ti,ab.
26   elder$.ti,ab.
27   geriatric$.ti,ab,hw.
28   senior$.ti,ab.
29   24 or 25 or 26 or 27 or 28
30   7 and 23 and 29
31   limit 30 to (clinical trial or controlled clinical trial or randomized controlled trial)
32   clinical trials/ or controlled clinical trials/ or randomized controlled trials/
33   double-blind method/ or random allocation/ or single-blind method/
34   random$.ti,ab.
35   32 or 33 or 34
36   30 and 35
37   31 or 36
38   limit 37 to english language

**Observational Studies of SSRI Harms**
Databse: PsycINFO and MEDLINE
Dates: 1988- December 2007
1    Antidepressive Agents, Second-Generation/
2    Serotonin Uptake Inhibitors/
3    ssri$.ti.
4    selective serotonin reuptake inhibitor$.ti.
5    antidepress$.ti.
6    (ssri$ or selective serotonin reuptake inhibitor$).ab.
7    5 and 6
8    1 or 2 or 3 or 4 or 7
9    suicide$.ti,ab,hw.
10   suicidal$.ti,ab,hw.
11   discontinu$.ti,ab,hw.
12   9 or 10 or 11
13   8 and 12
14   observational.ti,ab.
15   (cohort adj (study or studies)).ti,ab.
16   cohort analys$.ti,ab.
17   cohort studies/
18   retrospective$.ti,ab.
19   retrospective studies/
20   longitudinal$.ti,ab.
21   longitudinal studies/
22   (follow up adj (study or studies)).ti,ab.
23   follow-up studies/
24   prospective$.ti,ab.
25   prospective studies/
26   database$.ti,ab,hw.
27   nonrandomi$.ti,ab.
28   population$.ti,ab.
29   case control$.ti,ab.
30   case-control studies/
31   14 or 15 or 16 or 17 or 18 or 19 or 20 or 21 or 22 or 23 or 24 or 25 or 26 or 27 or 28 or 29 or 30
32   13 and 31
33   limit 32 to "all child (0 to 18 years)"
34   limit 32 to "all adult (19 plus years)"
35   33 not 34
36   32 not 35
37   limit 36 to (english language and yr="1988 - 2007")

**Appendix D Figure 2:** Screening Study Interventions and Approaches: Model for Inclusions and Exclusions

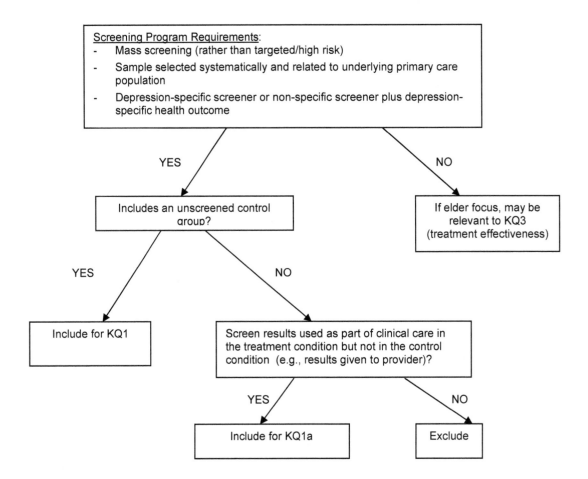

The 2002 USPSTF review took a broad approach to the evidence, considering trials that included both screening and additional support components to be relevant to the question of screening efficacy in addition to trials examining stand-alone screening programs. We have largely maintained this approach with some refinements in inclusion/exclusion criteria and in reporting. While the 2002 review included ten studies reporting health outcomes altogether, only five studies were also included in our review.[10,109-112] Of the five excluded studies, two were excluded because they did not meet our a priori quality standards, including a minimum of 4-week followup.[236,237] We excluded two other studies that did not use depression-specific screening instruments or report depression specific outcomes,[238,239] and one study that screened a high-risk population rather than a general population.[202]

The 2005 Cochrane review on this topic included four studies: two that we also included (both studies of elderly populations with negative outcomes) and two that we excluded due to lack of depression-specific measures, both also with negative findings. The Cochrane review specifically excluded studies that they judged to have extensive quality improvement components on the logic that it would be impossible to disentangle the effects of the screening component from those of the other intervention components. The Cochrane reviewer has noted in another published article that the UK National Screening Guidelines require screening alone to improve outcomes before recommending its use.[156] Thus, this approach is consistent with this requirement. Our conclusions are also consistent with this review's conclusions in that we did not find support for screening programs in any adult age range without additional care support components.

**Appendix F Table 1. Meta-analysis decision factors**

| Study Reference / Design | Newly identified cases only? | Unscreened control group? / Location and timing of screening? | Percent of screened patients who were positive for depression | Percent of patients currently or recently treated for depression at time of screen | Patient-level intervention beyond assessment and antidepressant medication? | Followup | Screening Instrument | Results, Primary Outcome / % control group in remission at followup |
|---|---|---|---|---|---|---|---|---|
| *Older Adults* | | | | | | | | |
| **Whooley** et al 2000[111] Cluster RCT | No | No, Waiting room, usually before visit | 14.1% positive | approx 20% used antidepressant in past 12 mos | Yes: series of 6 psycho-ed classes + 1 booster (but 12% pts attended) | 24-mo | GDS | No group differences in GDS; 50% remission @ 24 mos |
| **Bosmans** et al 2006[115] Cluster RCT | Yes | No, Before visit, presume waiting room | 14.7% positive | 0% currently treated | No | 12-mo | GDS | No group differences in MADRS score; 48% remission @ 12 mos |
| **Callahan** et al 1994[112] Cluster RCT | No | No, In exam room, during visit | 16.2% positive on CESD (first screener) 4.6% completed both screens, positive on both | approx 12% on antidepressant at baseline | Yes: educational materials, 3 depression-focused visits with provider | 6-mo | CESD + HAMD (2-step process) | No group differences on CESD; 12% responded @ 6 mo |
| **Rubenstein** et al 2007[116] | No | No, By mail | 41.0%, among those who met threshold for high risk for five conditions | NR | Yes: quarterly followup by case manager | 12-mo | GDS | I-group greater improvement in GDS (small effect); NR |
| *No focus on older adults* | | | | | | | | |
| **Williams** et al 1999[10] (low income) RCT | No | Yes, Waiting room, before appt. Also had research diagnostic interview w/in 2 wks of baseline appt. | 1-item screen: 41% pos CES-D: 33% pos | NR | No | 3-mo | CESD or 1-item | Mixed: no differences in % depressed but great % of I-group in full remission. Assessed via diagnostic interview; 27% remission @ 3 mos |
| **Wells** et al 2000[110] Cluster RCT | No | No, Waiting area, probably same day at appt, pts may have gotten results | 14.3% positive | NR | extensive | 6-mo, 12-mo, 57-mo | CIDI (2-step) | I-group better outcomes, % dep per CESD; 50% @ 6-mo |
| **Bergus** et al 2005[113] (rural) RCT | No | No, Waiting room, before visit | 13.8% positive | 38% on meds for dep OR anxiety, 60% history of tx for depression | No | 1-mo, 2.5-mo, 6-mo | PHQ-9 | No group diffs, change in PHQ, % remission; 38% remission @ 6 mos |

Screening for Depression in Adults

**Appendix F Table 1. Meta-analysis decision factors**

| Study Reference Design | Newly identified cases only? | Unscreened control group? Location and timing of screening? | Percent of screened patients who were positive for depression | Percent of patients currently or recently treated for depression at time of screen | Patient-level intervention beyond assessment and antidepressant medication? | Followup | Screening Instrument | Results, Primary Outcome % control group in remission at followup |
|---|---|---|---|---|---|---|---|---|
| **Jarjoura** et al 2004[114] (indigent) RCT | Yes | No Waiting room, before visit | 45.4% positive overall 9.2% positive AND not currently being treated for depression | 0% | minimal | 6-mo, 12-mo | BDI | I-group better outcomes, mixed model repeated measure BDI<br><br>21% showed ≥33% improvement in BDI score (avg of 6- and 12-mo scores) |
| **Rost** et al 2001[109] Cluster RCT | No, but only reported newly-identified and previously-identified cases separately | No Waiting room, before visit | 6.8% positive | ~44% overall | Yes, 8 weekly nurse education session, discuss treatment options, homework to enhance readiness to enage in treatment. | 6-mo | CIDI (2-step) | I-group better outcomes (change in CESD) **among newly identified cases only**<br><br>22% remission **among newly identified cases only** |

GDS=Geriatric Depression Scale; CESD=Center of Epidemiologic Studies Depression Scale; HAMD-Hamilton Depression Rating Scale; CIDI=Composite International Diagnostic Interview; PHQ-9=9-item Patient Health Questionnaire; BDI=Beck Depression Inventory

**Appendix G Table 1. Evidence table of screening trials-KQ1 and KQ1a.**

| Study / USPSTF Quality | Study design / Unit of randomization / Point of randomization / Setting | Intervention and control conditions | Depressive disorders identified or targeted / % Currently treated for depression | Location / Population targeted | CONSORT numbers | Population characteristics / Baseline depression scores | Inclusion and exclusion criteria |
|---|---|---|---|---|---|---|---|
| **KQ1 trial** | | | | | | | |
| Williams et al 1999[10]<br><br>Fair | RCT<br><br>Consecutive patients in study clinics recruited on designated days<br><br>Patients randomized before screen to longer screen, brief screen, or no screen. Diagnostic phone interview after visit.<br><br>Several different outpatient medical clinics | I1: Completed CES-D before scheduled appointment and results placed in chart on bright orange form (for everyone--not only positive screens)<br><br>I2: Same as above but used 1-item depression screen<br><br>C: Usual care (no screen)<br><br>All providers received guide for managing depression in primary care and continuing education session on interpreting case-finding questionnaire and diagnosing depression<br><br>All patients had post-visit diagnostic interview via phone | MDD, Dysthymia, Minor Depression<br><br>% Currently treated: NR | San Antonio, TX and Washington, D.C.<br><br>General outpatient primary care | 1,083 approached<br>1037 eligible<br>969 consented<br>969 screened<br>969 randomized<br><br>I1= 323<br>I2= 330<br>C= 316<br><br>863 complete baseline data<br>I1= 296<br>I2= 291<br>C= 276 | Mean Age:<br>I= 59<br>I= 58<br>C= 56<br><br>Female:<br>I1= 74%<br>I2= 68%<br>C: 71%<br><br>Hispanic:<br>I= 61%<br>I2= 59%<br>C= 58%<br><br>Black:<br>I1= 9%<br>I2= 12%<br>C= 10%<br><br>Yrs educations:<br>I1= 10<br>I2= 11<br>C= 11<br><br>% income <$7,200:<br>I1=42%; I2=40%;<br>C=36%<br>% income ≥ $16,800<br>I1=24%; I2=25%;<br>C=24%<br><br>% any depression diagnosis: I1=12.4%;<br>I2=13.8%; C=13.8% | Inclusion: scheduled appt at one of study clinics<br><br>Exclusion: No telephone; no stable address |

USPSTF=United States Preventive Services Task Force; AHRQ=Agency for Healthcare Research Quality; RCT=Randomized Control Trial; CES-D=Center for Epidemiologic Studies Depression Scale; I=Intervention; C=Control; MDD=Major Depressive Disorder; NR=Not Reported; AE=Adverse Events; PRIME-MD=Primary Care Evaluation of Mental Disorders; SES=Socio-Economic Status; GDS=Geriatric Depression Scale; GP=General Practitioner; GPSS=Geriatric Postal Screening Survey; PHQ-9=Patient Health Questionnaire; NS=Not Specified; BDI=Beck's Depression Inventory; SF-36=Short Form; WHO-CIDI=World Health Organization Composite International Diagnostic Interview; QI=Quality Improvement; CBT=Cognitive Behavioral Therapy; HAM-D=Hamilton Rating Scale for Depression; SIP=Sickness Impact Profile; MADRS=Montgomery Asberg Depression Rating Scale

Screening for Depression in Adults

**Appendix G Table 1. Evidence table of screening trials-KQ1 and KQ1a.**

| Study<br>USPSTF Quality | Screening instrument<br>Mode of administration<br>Who administered and scored<br>How results sent to clinician<br>Diagnostic work-up | Follow-up | Outcomes<br>Depression outcomes<br>Other health outcomes<br>Adverse events | Group selected for analysis<br>Similarity to all randomized<br>Similarity at baseline | Analysis | Results<br>P values<br>NS=p>0.05,<br>*p< 0.05,<br>**p<0.01 | Comments |
|---|---|---|---|---|---|---|---|
| **KQ1 trial** | | | | | | | |
| Williams et al 1999[10]<br><br>Fair | I1: CES-D, I2: "Have you felt depressed or sad much of the time in the past year?"<br><br>Paper-and-pencil, in medical clinic before appointment<br><br>Who administered/scored: NR<br><br>Results placed in chart on bright orange sheet of paper<br><br>Patient contacted by phone by the researcher after visit to complete diagnostic interview for DSM-IIIR diagnosis | 3-month, San Antonio clinics only. Only followed up patients with diagnosis confirmed by post-visit phone interview + random sample of non-depressed per phone interview | Depression: % depressed; % ≤1 DSM-IIIR depression symptoms<br><br>Other: None<br><br>AE: NR | Only those in follow-up group (see follow-up time frame)<br><br>NR<br><br>NR | Combined I1 & I2; Compared I vs. C on % depressed, % ≤1 DSM-R, # depressive symptoms. Specific test NR. | % Depressed @ 3-mo (of all followed-up): I=37% (56/153) C=46% (30/65) p=0.19<br><br>% Recovered (of those with depression diagnosis per post-visit phone interview)*: I=48% (32/67) C=27% (8/30) p<0.05<br><br>Mean symptom count reduction: I=1.6, C=1.5 p=0.21<br><br>Results similar when only analyzed those who had followup (not sure how missings handled above) | San Antonio clinics only. Only followed up patients with diagnosis confirmed by post-visit phone interview + random sample of non-depressed per phone interview |

USPSTF=United States Preventive Services Task Force; AHRQ=Agency for Healthcare Research Quality; RCT=Randomized Control Trial; CES-D=Center for Epidemiologic Studies Depression Scale; I=Intervention; C=Control; MDD=Major Depressive Disorder; NR=Not Reported; AE=Adverse Events; PRIME-MD=Primary Care Evaluation of Mental Disorders; SES=Socio-Economic Status; GDS=Geriatric Depression Scale; GP=General Practitioner; GPSS=Geriatric Postal Screening Survey; PHQ-9=Patient Health Questionnaire; NS=Not Specified; BDI=Beck's Depression Inventory; SF-36=Short Form; WHO-CIDI=World Health Organization Composite International Diagnostic Interview; QI=Quality Improvement; CBT=Cognitive Behavioral Therapy; HAM-D=Hamilton Rating Scale for Depression; SIP=Sickness Impact Profile; MADRS=Montgomery Asberg Depression Rating Scale

Screening for Depression in Adults

**Appendix G Table 1. Evidence table of screening trials-KQ1 and KQ1a.**

| Study<br><br>USPSTF Quality | Study design<br>Unit of randomization<br>Point of randomization<br>Setting | Intervention and control conditions | Depressive disorders identified or targeted<br><br>% Currently treated for depression | Location<br><br>Population targeted | CONSORT numbers | Population characteristics<br><br>Baseline depression scores | Inclusion and exclusion criteria |
|---|---|---|---|---|---|---|---|
| **KQ1a trials** | | | | | | | |
| Bosmans et al 2006[115]<br><br>Fair | RCT, cluster randomized at clinic level<br><br>Randomized before screen, enrolled if positive screen + diagnosis confirmed by PRIME-MD<br><br>General practice | I: Screening; further evaluation by provider to determine if meet MDD criteria using PRIME-MD; providers attend 4-hr training session on screening, diagnosis, and treatment of late-life depression. Two treatment phases: every 2 wks for 2 months; monthly for 4 months.<br><br>C: Screening, further evaluation by study staff to determine if meet MDD criteria using PRIME-MD. Practitioner remained blinded to results; no training. | MDD<br><br>0% currently using antidepressants | Amsterdam, The Netherlands<br><br>Older (age 55+) general practice patients | 3,937 screened<br>579 pos screen<br>339 agree to diagnostic interview<br>178 MDD diagnosis<br>145 consent to rest of study<br><br>I=70; C=75<br><br>I=18 clinics; C=16 clinics | Mean Age:<br>I=66.4; C= 64.7<br><br>Female:<br>I=66%; C=54%<br><br>Race: NR<br><br>SES: NR<br><br>100% not on antidepressants<br><br>History of depression:<br>I=85%; C=82% | Inclusion: age 55+; visit with general practitioner; GDS-15 score ≥5; PRIME-MD diagnosis of MDD;<br><br>Exclusion: current use of antidepressants; current psychosis; bipolar, or drug abuse diagnosis; severe social dysfunction; inability to communicate in Dutch; impaired cognitive functioning |
| Bergus et al 2005[113]<br><br>Fair | RCT; randomized at patient level<br>Randomized using random number table after positive screen, all randomized<br>Two screened<br>private rural family practice clinics with 10 physicians | I: Provider asked to review PHQ-9 results, educated about PHQ-9C: Providers educated about PHQ-9, did not receive screen results | Accepted all positive screens, used screen cut-offs to categorize as Major and Minor depression for sub-analyses 38% on medications for depression or anxiety | Iowa; ruralGeneral outpatient family practice | 951 approached861 completed screen119 positive screen59 enrolledI=27; C=33 | Mean age: I=38.2; C=43.4<br>Female: I=62%;C=70%<br>Caucasian: I=92%; C=96%<br>Some college: I=58%, C=44%<br>History of depression treatment: 60%<br>Currently treated for depression: 38%<br>PHQ: I=12.0; C=12.7<br>All baseline differences-NS | Inclusion: English-speaking; adult; patient at study clinicExclusion: dementia |

USPSTF=United States Preventive Services Task Force; AHRQ=Agency for Healthcare Research Quality; RCT=Randomized Control Trial; CES-D=Center for Epidemiologic Studies Depression Scale; I=Intervention; C=Control; MDD=Major Depressive Disorder; NR=Not Reported; AE=Adverse Events; PRIME-MD=Primary Care Evaluation of Mental Disorders; SES=Socio-Economic Status; GDS=Geriatric Depression Scale; GP=General Practitioner; GPSS=Geriatric Postal Screening Survey; PHQ-9=Patient Health Questionnaire; NS=Not Specified; BDI=Beck's Depression Inventory; SF-36=Short Form; WHO-CIDI=World Health Organization Composite International Diagnostic Interview; QI=Quality Improvement; CBT=Cognitive Behavioral Therapy; HAM-D=Hamilton Rating Scale for Depression; SIP=Sickness Impact Profile; MADRS=Montgomery Asberg Depression Rating Scale

Screening for Depression in Adults

**Appendix G Table 1. Evidence table of screening trials-KQ1 and KQ1a.**

| Study USPSTF Quality | Screening instrument Mode of administration Who administered and scored How results sent to clinician Diagnostic work-up | Follow-up | Outcomes Depression outcomes Other health outcomes Adverse events | Group selected for analysis Similarity to all randomized Similarity at baseline | Analysis | Results P values NS=p>0.05, *p< 0.05, **p<0.01 | Comments |
|---|---|---|---|---|---|---|---|
| **KQ1a trials** | | | | | | | |
| Bosmans et al 2006[115]  Fair | GDS, PRIME-MD GDS mode NR, PRIME-MD interview  I: GP assistant admin and score GDS, GP admin/score PRIME-MD  C: research assistant admin and score both GDS and PRIME-MD. Result given to GP, GP administer PRIME-MD if screened positive.  Validation through GP or research assistant administration of PRIME-MD | 12-months | Depression: MDD diagnosis from PRIME-MD; depression severity from MADRS  Other: Quality Adjusted Life Years from EuroQol (EQ-5D)  AE: NR | Completing follow-up assessment (86% of enrolled)  NR  Enrolled group similar on age, sex, marital status, previous history of depression, and baseline depression severity | t-test for depression severity and QALYs, Chi-sq for percent recovered  Intention to treat on all who completed all followup. | % recovered: I=43%; C=48%, p=0.60 Mean change in MADRS from baseline: I=-7.8; C=-7.2, p=0.70 Mean QALYs gained: I=0.65; C=0.70, p=0.20 Analysis on I=58; C=67 | |
| Bergus et al 2005[113]  Fair | PHQ-9Mode: NRAdmin/score: NR 1Provider asked to review completed PHQ-9Validation: provider review | 4-, 10-, 24-week | Depression: Change in PHQ-9 score; remission per PHQ-9Other: noneAE: NR | Completed ≥1 followup (inferred). Those unable to be contacted were dropped from the studyNRyes | t-tests; repeated measures ANOVA for continuous measuresChi-sq for % remissionPHQ9 scores carried forward for missing data | 10 week followupAll subjects: Change in PHQ: I= -5.8; C= -5.8 (p=0.45)% Remission: I=54%; C=37% (p=0.35) Patient with Major Depression:Change in PHQ: I= -7.3; C= -9.1 (NS)% Remission: I= 36%; C= 38% (NS) 24 week followup All subjects: Change in PHQ: I= -5.7; C= -5.0 (p=0.45)% Remission: I=52%; C=38% (p=0.35) Patient with Major Depression: Change in PHQ: I= -8.5; C= -8.2 (NS)% Remission: I= 54%; C= 31% (NS) | Small N, probable contamination, blinding NR |

Screening for Depression in Adults

**Appendix G Table 1. Evidence table of screening trials–KQ1 and KQ1a.**

| Study<br><br>USPSTF Quality | Study design<br>Unit of randomization<br>Point of randomization<br>Setting | Intervention and control conditions | Depressive disorders identified or targeted<br><br>% Currently treated for depression | Location<br><br>Population targeted | CONSORT numbers | Population characteristics<br><br>Baseline depression scores | Inclusion and exclusion criteria |
|---|---|---|---|---|---|---|---|
| **KQ1a trials** | | | | | | | |
| Jarjoura 2004[114]<br><br>Fair | RCT; randomized at patient level<br><br>Randomized by permuted blocks of 40 using sealed envelopes after positive screen; all randomized screened<br><br>Indigent primary care clinic | I: Screening nurse gave results + treatment protocol to provider. Protocol includes: explore symptoms to confirm diagnosis; rule out other explanations for positive screen; educate patient & give materials; offer appointment for behavioral counseling; prescribe antidepressant if acceptable to patient; schedule return visit in 4 weeks<br><br>C: provider not informed of results; patient told may have problem with depression and that there are effective treatments | Not specified–just positive screen<br><br>0% currently being treated for depression | Ohio<br><br>Internal medicine residency clinic | 1,095 screened<br>497 positive screen<br>101 not currently treated for depression<br>61 randomized*<br>I=33; C=28<br><br>*24 of those not randomized were ineligible due to suicidal ideation | Mean Age: I=45; C=46<br><br>Female: I=76%; C=61%<br>Race: NR<br>SES: NR, but all were required to be below federal poverty level.<br><br>100% not current treatment for depression<br><br>BDI: 28 (I) 23 (C)<br><br>All characteristics-NS | Inclusion: age 18+; Medicaid or low-income & no private insurance; positive screen for major depression episode; **not receiving treatment for depression**; not seeking help for depression or other emotional problems; could read and respond to questionnaire<br><br>Exclusion: suicidal ideation |

USPSTF=United States Preventive Services Task Force; AHRQ=Agency for Healthcare Research Quality; RCT=Randomized Control Trial; CES-D=Center for Epidemiologic Studies Depression Scale; I=Intervention; C=Control; MDD=Major Depressive Disorder; NR=Not Reported; AE=Adverse Events; PRIME-MD=Primary Care Evaluation of Mental Disorders; SES=Socio-Economic Status; GDS=Geriatric Depression Scale; GP=General Practitioner; GPSS=Geriatric Postal Screening Survey; PHQ-9=Patient Health Questionnaire; NS=Not Specified; BDI=Beck's Depression Inventory; SF-36=Short Form; WHO-CIDI=World Health Organization Composite International Diagnostic Interview; QI=Quality Improvement; CBT=Cognitive Behavioral Therapy; HAM-D=Hamilton Rating Scale for Depression; SIP=Sickness Impact Profile; MADRS=Montgomery Asberg Depression Rating Scale

Screening for Depression in Adults

**Appendix G Table 1. Evidence table of screening trials-KQ1 and KQ1a.**

| Study<br><br>USPSTF Quality | Screening instrument<br>Mode of administration<br>Who administered and scored<br>How results sent to clinician<br>Diagnostic work-up | Follow-up | Outcomes<br>Depression outcomes<br>Other health outcomes<br>Adverse events | Group selected for analysis<br>Similarity to all randomized<br>Similarity at baseline | Analysis | Results<br>P values<br>NS=p>0.05,<br>*p< 0.05,<br>**p<0.01 | Comments |
|---|---|---|---|---|---|---|---|
| **KQ1a trials** | | | | | | | |
| Jarjoura 2004[114]<br><br>Fair | PRIME-MD<br><br>Presume mode paper-and-pencil, based on reading requirement<br><br>Nurse administered/score<br><br>Nurse gave results to clinician<br><br>Provider asked to validate screen results | 6-, 12-month | Depression: BDI, PRIME-MD (1-yr only)<br><br>Other: utilization of medical & behavioral services, costs of care, SF-36<br><br>AE: NR | Complete ≥1 followup (inferred)<br><br>NR<br><br>NR | Repeated measures mixed model.<br><br>Adjusted for baseline | % showing ≥33% decline in BDI (averaging 6- and 12-mo data):<br>39% (I), 21% (C) (p NR)<br><br>6-mo: I-group BDI change 7.6 pts > C-group change (p NR)<br>12-mo: I-group BDI change 6.5 pts > C-group change (p=0.03)<br><br>SF-36 QOL "Intervention effect"=3.6 (p=0.27)<br><br>Health Care costs NS (p-value range 0.26 - 0.93) | Small **N**, probable contamination, control group told test results, possibly capitalizing on regression to mean since I-group 6 patients higher on BDI at baseline (though NS)<br><br>Only newly-detected depression |

USPSTF=United States Preventive Services Task Force; AHRQ=Agency for Healthcare Research Quality; RCT=Randomized Control Trial; CES-D=Center for Epidemiologic Studies Depression Scale; I=Intervention; C=Control; MDD=Major Depressive Disorder; NR=Not Reported; AE=Adverse Events; PRIME-MD=Primary Care Evaluation of Mental Disorders; SES=Socio-Economic Status; GDS=Geriatric Depression Scale; GP=General Practitioner; GPSS=Geriatric Postal Screening Survey; PHQ-9=Patient Health Questionnaire; NS=Not Specified; BDI=Beck's Depression Inventory; SF-36=Short Form; WHO-CIDI=World Health Organization Composite International Diagnostic Interview; QI=Quality Improvement; CBT=Cognitive Behavioral Therapy; HAM-D=Hamilton Rating Scale for Depression; SIP=Sickness Impact Profile; MADRS=Montgomery Asberg Depression Rating Scale

Screening for Depression in Adults

**Appendix G Table 1. Evidence table of screening trials-KQ1 and KQ1a.**

| Study<br><br>USPSTF Quality | Study design<br>Unit of randomization<br>Point of randomization<br>Setting | Intervention and control conditions | Depressive disorders identified or targeted<br><br>% Currently treated for depression | Location<br><br>Population targeted | CONSORT numbers | Population characteristics<br><br>Baseline depression scores | Inclusion and exclusion criteria |
|---|---|---|---|---|---|---|---|
| **KQ1a trials** | | | | | | | |
| Rost et al 2001[109]<br><br>Rost et al 2000[190]<br><br>Rost et al, 2006[119]<br><br>Rost et al, 2005[174]<br><br>Good | RCT, cluster randomized<br><br>Randomized 12 matched primary care practices, 6 to each condition<br><br>one control-group practice did not meet recruitment goals and so was replaced with another practice; participant enrolled after 2-step screen process, if patient positive on both screens | I: 2 physicians, 2 nurses, 1 administrative person trained; administrative staff recruited participant before index visit with physician; if physician confirm diagnosis, patient scheduled return visit in 1 week; re-assessed immediately before 1-week visit, patient educated about preferred treatment; ask patient to complete homework assignments; arranged further follow-up; up to 9 weekly visits with same pattern<br><br>C: Administrative staff administered screening, but physicians were not informed which patients were participating and nurses did not meet with depressed patients. | Major Depression<br><br>I: 48%; C: 40% recently (past 6 months) treated for depression | CO, MI, MN, NJ, NC, ND, OK, OR, VA, WI, urban and rural | 11,006 approached 9,555 completed 1st step screen 2,082 positive 1st step screen 653 positive 2nd step screen 479 patients enrolled I=239; C=240<br><br>Patients with 6-mo followup: Previously-known cases N=243, Newly-identified cases N=189 | Mean age: I=41.4; C=43.9<br><br>Female: I=84%; C=84%<br>Caucasian: I=84%; C=84%<br>High school: I=79%; C= 79%<br><br>PHQ: I=12.0; C=12.7 all baseline differences NS | Inclusion: routine-length appt with participating provider; age 18+; sufficient English literacy/cog. function to complete questionnaire; no acute life-threatening physical condition; access to telephone; positive score on both screening instruments;<br><br>Exclusion: pregnant, breastfeeding, or < 3 mos post-partum; bereavement; did not intend to receive on-going care in target clinic during next 12 months; lifetime history of mania; use of lithium; current alcohol dependence |

Screening for Depression in Adults

# Appendix G Table 1. Evidence table of screening trials-KQ1 and KQ1a.

| Study<br><br>USPSTF Quality | Screening instrument<br>Mode of administration<br>Who administered and scored<br>How results sent to clinician<br>Diagnostic work-up | Follow-up | Outcomes<br>Depression outcomes<br>Other health outcomes<br>Adverse events | Group selected for analysis<br>Similarity to all randomized<br>Similarity at baseline | Analysis | Results<br>P values<br>NS=p>0.05,<br>*p< 0.05,<br>**p<0.01 | Comments |
|---|---|---|---|---|---|---|---|
| **KQ1a trials** | | | | | | | |
| Rost et al 2001[109]<br><br>Rost et al 2000[190]<br><br>Rost et al, 2006[119]<br><br>Rost et al, 2005[174]<br><br>Good | (1) 2 WHO-CIDI items<br>(2) 9-item Inventory to Diagnose Depression<br><br>Mode: NR<br><br>Office staff hand-scored<br><br>Note placed in front of chart informing provider that the patient had screened positive for MDD and agreed to be in the study<br><br>Provider asked to evaluate depression diagnosis and begin study protocol of agreed with diagnosis | 6-month on everyone; 12-month, 18-month, 24-month only on those with newly-identified depression episode | Depression: CES-D collected via phone interview<br><br>Other: SF-36<br><br>AE: None | Completed the follow-up interview. Report separately those who had been treated for depression in past 6 months and those who had not.<br><br>NR<br><br>NR | Intention-to-treat hierarchical models stratified by whether patient had recently been treated for depression, controlling for all baseline differences that were p<0.20 | Decrease in CES-D baseline to 6-mo: Recently treated: I=14.5; C= 11.0<br><br>Newly identified depression: I=21.7; C=13.5*<br><br>% Remission at 24 mos (CES-D≥15) in newly identified depression only: I=74%; C=41% | No overall results reported, only by subgroups of whether they had been in treatment for depression at baseline or not. Overall differences WERE significant, per personal communication (Rost, 2006) |

USPSTF=United States Preventive Services Task Force; AHRQ=Agency for Healthcare Research Quality; RCT=Randomized Control Trial; CES-D=Center for Epidemiologic Studies Depression Scale; I=Intervention; C=Control; MDD=Major Depressive Disorder; NR=Not Reported; AE=Adverse Events; PRIME-MD=Primary Care Evaluation of Mental Disorders; SES=Socio-Economic Status; GDS=Geriatric Depression Scale; GP=General Practitioner; GPSS=Geriatric Postal Screening Survey; PHQ-9=Patient Health Questionnaire; NS=Not Specified; BDI=Beck's Depression Inventory; SF-36=Short Form; WHO-CIDI=World Health Organization Composite International Diagnostic Interview; QI=Quality Improvement; CBT=Cognitive Behavioral Therapy; HAM-D=Hamilton Rating Scale for Depression; SIP=Sickness Impact Profile; MADRS=Montgomery Asberg Depression Rating Scale

Screening for Depression in Adults

**Appendix G Table 1. Evidence table of screening trials-KQ1 and KQ1a.**

| Study<br><br>USPSTF Quality | Study design<br>Unit of randomization<br>Point of randomization<br>Setting | Intervention and control conditions | Depressive disorders identified or targeted<br><br>% Currently treated for depression | Location<br><br>Population targeted | CONSORT numbers | Population characteristics<br><br>Baseline depression scores | Inclusion and exclusion criteria |
|---|---|---|---|---|---|---|---|
| **KQ1a trials** | | | | | | | |
| Whooley et al 2000[111]<br><br>Fair | RCT, randomized at clinic level<br><br>Randomized before screen, all randomized screened<br><br>Primary care | I: provider notified of screening results + handout with score interpretation and general recommendations; group psycho-education classes offered to patients and family; 1-hour provider training on depression management<br><br>C: screening & no feedback, 1-hour provider training on depression management | Not specified-just positive screen<br><br>% on antidepressants in past 12 month: I=23%, C=17% | Oakland, CA<br><br>Geriatric (65+) outpatient primary care | # approached NR<br>2,896 eligible for screening<br>2,346 screened<br>2,346 randomized<br>331 positive screen<br><br>I=162<br>C=169 | Mean age: I=75.7; C=75.9<br><br>Female: I=59%; C=62%<br>African American: I=28%; C=37%<br>Caucasian: I=49%; C=39%<br>Completed High School: I=87%; C=76% (p=0.04) | Inclusion: age 65+, had medical appointment at one of study clinics<br><br>Exclusion: NR |

USPSTF=United States Preventive Services Task Force; AHRQ=Agency for Healthcare Research Quality; RCT=Randomized Control Trial; CES-D=Center for Epidemiologic Studies Depression Scale; I=Intervention; C=Control; MDD=Major Depressive Disorder; NR=Not Reported; AE=Adverse Events; PRIME-MD=Primary Care Evaluation of Mental Disorders; SES=Socio-Economic Status; GDS=Geriatric Depression Scale; GP=General Practitioner; GPSS=Geriatric Postal Screening Survey; PHQ-9=Patient Health Questionnaire; NS=Not Specified; BDI=Beck's Depression Inventory; SF-36=Short Form; WHO-CIDI=World Health Organization Composite International Diagnostic Interview; QI=Quality Improvement; CBT=Cognitive Behavioral Therapy; HAM-D=Hamilton Rating Scale for Depression; SIP=Sickness Impact Profile; MADRS=Montgomery Asberg Depression Rating Scale

Screening for Depression in Adults

**Appendix G Table 1. Evidence table of screening trials-KQ1 and KQ1a.**

| Study<br>USPSTF Quality | Screening instrument<br>Mode of administration<br>Who administered and scored<br>How results sent to clinician<br>Diagnostic work-up | Follow-up | Outcomes<br>Depression outcomes<br>Other health outcomes<br>Adverse events | Group selected for analysis<br>Similarity to all randomized<br>Similarity at baseline | Analysis | Results<br>P values<br>NS=p>0.05,<br>*p< 0.05,<br>**p<0.01 | Comments |
|---|---|---|---|---|---|---|---|
| **KQ1a trials** | | | | | | | |
| Whooley et al 2000[111]<br><br>Fair | GDS<br><br>Mode: NR<br><br>Administered/scored: research assistant<br><br>Results + explanatory hand-out put in chart<br><br>Validation at discretion of provider | 2-year | Depression: GDS; % depressed<br><br>Other: # visits; hospitalization<br><br>AE: NR | Baseline GDS≥6: N=331 (I=162; C=169)<br>2-year GDS only avail for I=97, C=109<br><br>Those completing 2 yr followup were more likely to be divorced/separated and had fewer clinic visits in previous 12 mo.<br><br>Similar on all variables reported except % completed high school (p=0.04, fewer in C group) and income category (p=0.002, C group lower income, fewer unknown income) | Mean change based on stepwise regression-include all baseline demographic/social/health variables, Keeping variables with p≤0.05 in model;<br>Chi-sq of % improved; logistic of # improved, controlling for baseline differences;<br>Compare differences in mean # clinic visits and hospitalizations | GDS: both groups significant change over time; no group differences<br><br>% depressed: no group differences<br>I=42% (41/97); C=50% (54/109)<br><br>Adjusted mean decrease in GDS score from baseline: I=1.8; C=2.2 (p=0.41)<br><br>Health care utilization: no group differences<br># clinic visits: I=1.8; C=1.6<br># hospitalizations: I=1.1; C=1.0 | Only analyzed those who screened positive at baseline<br><br>12% attended group session. |

USPSTF=United States Preventive Services Task Force; AHRQ=Agency for Healthcare Research Quality; RCT=Randomized Control Trial; CES-D=Center for Epidemiologic Studies Depression Scale; I=Intervention; C=Control; MDD=Major Depressive Disorder; NR=Not Reported; AE=Adverse Events; PRIME-MD=Primary Care Evaluation of Mental Disorders; SES=Socio-Economic Status; GDS=Geriatric Depression Scale; GP=General Practitioner; GPSS=Geriatric Postal Screening Survey; PHQ-9=Patient Health Questionnaire; NS=Not Specified; BDI=Beck's Depression Inventory; SF-36=Short Form; WHO-CIDI=World Health Organization Composite International Diagnostic Interview; QI=Quality Improvement; CBT=Cognitive Behavioral Therapy; HAM-D=Hamilton Rating Scale for Depression; SIP=Sickness Impact Profile; MADRS=Montgomery Asberg Depression Rating Scale

Screening for Depression in Adults

**Appendix G Table 1. Evidence table of screening trials-KQ1 and KQ1a.**

| Study / USPSTF Quality | Study design / Unit of randomization / Point of randomization / Setting | Intervention and control conditions | Depressive disorders identified or targeted / % Currently treated for depression | Location / Population targeted | CONSORT numbers | Population characteristics / Baseline depression scores | Inclusion and exclusion criteria |
|---|---|---|---|---|---|---|---|
| **KQ1a trial** | | | | | | | |
| Wells et al 2000[110] Wells et al 2004[118] Sherbourne et al 2001[169] Rubenstein et al, 1999[240] Good | RCT, cluster randomized Randomized managed care organization regions; regions in matched clusters of 3, each cluster had a region assigned to one of 3 conditions; individual provider consented to participate or not. Consecutive patients in study clinics screened, only positive screen enrolled Primary care | I1: (QI-Meds) Screening; institutional monetary commitment; staff and clinician training (1- or 2-day workshops); clinician manuals; monthly training lectures; academic detailing as needed; numerous materials for clinicians, staff, patients; trained nurse specialists for followup assessment and on-going adherence support (medication adherence, presumably) I2: (QI-Therapy) Screening; same QI elements as above except trained therapists to provide individual or group manualized CBT and reduced co-pay for therapy rather than nurse med specialists C: Screening; participant told they could inform their providers of screen results; medical directors mailed the AHRQ depression practice guidelines + quick reference guides for clinicians | MDD and Dysthymia-specific screener used % Currently treated: NR | 7 geographic regions-sites chosen to oversample Mexican Americans Outpatient primary care | 44,052 approached 37,452 consent to screening 27,332 screened* 3,918 positive screen 2,176 eligible for enrollment 1,356 patients enrolled (46 clinics randomized) I=913 (30 clinics); C=443 (16 clinics) *most of those not screened were ineligible because they were not patients of study providers | Mean age: I=44.5; C=42.2 Female: I=71.6%; C=69.0% Hispanic: I=29.1%; C=30.6% Caucasian: I=57.9%; C= 55.3% Completed college: I=22.2%; C=15.0% (p=0.001) % depressed per baseline CES-D: I=75.4; C= 75.7% | Inclusion: positive screen; intended to use clinic as source of care for next 12 months Exclusion: <18; acute medical emergency; did not speak English or Spanish; no insurance or public-pay arrangement that covered mental health care |

USPSTF=United States Preventive Services Task Force; AHRQ=Agency for Healthcare Research Quality; RCT=Randomized Control Trial; CES-D=Center for Epidemiologic Studies Depression Scale; I=Intervention; C=Control; MDD=Major Depressive Disorder; NR=Not Reported; AE=Adverse Events; PRIME-MD=Primary Care Evaluation of Mental Disorders; SES=Socio-Economic Status; GDS=Geriatric Depression Scale; GP=General Practitioner; GPSS=Geriatric Postal Screening Survey; PHQ-9=Patient Health Questionnaire; NS=Not Specified; BDI=Beck's Depression Inventory; SF-36=Short Form; WHO-CIDI=World Health Organization Composite International Diagnostic Interview; QI=Quality Improvement; CBT=Cognitive Behavioral Therapy; HAM-D=Hamilton Rating Scale for Depression; SIP=Sickness Impact Profile; MADRS=Montgomery Asberg Depression Rating Scale

Screening for Depression in Adults

**Appendix G Table 1. Evidence table of screening trials-KQ1 and KQ1a.**

| Study / USPSTF Quality | Screening instrument / Mode of administration / Who administered and scored / How results sent to clinician / Diagnostic work-up | Follow-up | Outcomes / Depression outcomes / Other health outcomes / Adverse events | Group selected for analysis / Similarity to all randomized / Similarity at baseline | Analysis | Results / P values / NS=p>0.05, *p< 0.05, **p<0.01 | Comments |
|---|---|---|---|---|---|---|---|
| **KQ1a trials** | | | | | | | |
| Wells et al 2000[110]<br><br>Wells et al 2004[118]<br><br>Sherbourne et al 2001[189]<br><br>Rubenstein et al, 1999[240]<br><br>Good | CIDI-MDD and dysthymia sections (based on DSM)<br><br>Mode: NR<br><br>Administered/scored: study staff<br><br>Intervention clinics provided lists of study participants. Control clinics not notified. | 6-month, 12-month, 18-month, 24-month, 57-month<br><br>6-24-month follow-up from mailed questionnaire with phone follow-up, 57-month followup by phone | Depression: CES-D; % probably MDD or dysthymia diagnosis per CIDI<br><br>Other: SF-12 Mental health and physical summary scales<br><br>AE: NR | Those completing follow-up qx 6-mo N=1,156 (85%), 12-mo N=1,126 (83%) 24-mo N=NR 57-mo N=924 (73%)<br><br>NR<br><br>I slightly older and more likely to be married than C | Patient-level intention-to-treat, using multiple imputation for missing data at item-level. Intraclass correlations were close to zero so analyses were not adjusted for cluster effects.<br><br>Multivariate regression models | % depression per CES-D cut-off Baseline: I=75.4; C= 75.7 6-month: I=55.4; C=64.4** 12-month: I=54.5; C=61.4*<br><br>Still positive on CIDI: 6-month: I=39.9%; C=49.9** 12-month: I=41.6%; C=51.2** 24-month: I=est 35%; C=34% 57-month: I=37.0%; C=43.6%*<br><br>Mean mental health summary score: Baseline: I=35.6; C=36.1 6-month: I=41.6; C=39.8** 12-month: I=40.9; C=39.3* 57-month: I=44.8; C=42.6<br><br>Mean physical summary score Baseline: I=45.2; C=44.6 6-month: I=43.9; C=43.7 12-month: I=44.1; C=44.6<br><br>Depression diagnosis per CIDI interview (24-month) I1=39%; I2=31%; C=34% | Fairly extensive baseline data collection procedures for all participants, plus ma led followup questionnaire every 6 months |

USPSTF=United States Preventive Services Task Force; AHRQ=Agency for Healthcare Research Quality; RCT=Randomized Control Trial; CES-D=Center for Epidemiologic Studies Depression Scale; I=Intervention; C=Control; MDD=Major Depressive Disorder; NR=Not Reported; AE=Adverse Events; PRIME-MD=Primary Care Evaluation of Mental Disorders; SES=Socio-Economic Status; GDS=Geriatric Depression Scale; GP=General Practitioner; GPSS=Geriatric Postal Screening Survey; PHQ-9=Patient Health Questionnaire; NS=Not Specified; BDI=Beck's Depression Inventory; SF-36=Short Form; WHO-CIDI=World Health Organization Composite International Diagnostic Interview; QI=Quality Improvement; CBT=Cognitive Behavioral Therapy; HAM-D=Hamilton Rating Scale for Depression; SIP=Sickness Impact Profile; MADRS=Montgomery Asberg Depression Rating Scale

Screening for Depression in Adults

103

**Appendix G Table 1. Evidence table of screening trials-KQ1 and KQ1a.**

| Study<br><br>USPSTF Quality | Study design<br>Point of randomization<br>Unit of randomization<br>Setting | Intervention and control conditions | Depressive disorders identified or targeted<br><br>% Currently treated for depression | Location<br><br>Population targeted | CONSORT numbers | Population characteristics<br><br>Baseline depression scores | Inclusion and exclusion criteria |
|---|---|---|---|---|---|---|---|
| **KQ1a trial** | | | | | | | |
| Callahan et al 1994[112]<br><br>Fair | RCT<br><br>Clinical practice sessions randomized, patients scheduled during selected practice sessions and who screened positive in two separate interviews were enrolled.<br><br>Primary care | I: 2-step screen; 3 appointments with primary provider over 3 months to address symptoms of depression; letter for provider including HAM-D results, medications associated with depression, and treatment recommendations placed in chart; educational materials for patient included in chart; post-visit questionnaire<br><br>C: 2-step screen; no screening results given to provider; further appointments at discretion of provider; post-visit provider questionnaire for baseline interview visit<br><br>Other: N=97 randomly selected for extensive psychiatric interview for other purposes, not included in these results<br><br>All providers given talk on late-life treatment of depression; any patient positive for suicidal ideation at baseline interview referred for immediate psych evaluation | Not specified-just positive screen<br><br>% on antidepressants: I=10.0%; C=13.5% (NS) | Indiana, multi-specialty ambulatory care clinic associated with urban county hospital<br><br>Target age 60+ | 4,413 approached<br>3,767 screened during primary care visit for depression, alcohol, & dementia<br>612 positive CES-D<br>515 retained (randomly selected 97 for other purposes, not included in this study)<br>254 consented to 2nd interview<br>175 positive on HAM-D<br>175 enrolled<br>I=100; C=75 | Mean age I=65.5; C=65.1<br><br>Female: I=76.0%; C=75.7%<br><br>African American: I=50.0%; C=52.7%<br><br>Years of education: I=8.6; C=9.1<br><br>Mean HAM-D: I=22.0; C=21.8<br><br>Mean SIP: I=33.0; C=29.9<br><br>No statistical differences | Inclusion: age 60+; regularly-scheduled primary care visit; score ≥16 on CES-D; score ≥15 on HAM-D<br><br>Exclusion: prisoners; patients residing in nursing home, unable to speak English; hearing impaired |

USPSTF=United States Preventive Services Task Force; AHRQ=Agency for Healthcare Research Quality; RCT=Randomized Control Trial; CES-D=Center for Epidemiologic Studies Depression Scale; I=Intervention; C=Control; MDD=Major Depressive Disorder; NR=Not Reported; AE=Adverse Events; PRIME-MD=Primary Care Evaluation of Mental Disorders; SES=Socio-Economic Status; GDS=Geriatric Depression Scale; GP=General Practitioner; GPSS=Geriatric Postal Screening Survey; PHQ-9=Patient Health Questionnaire; NS=Not Specified; BDI=Beck's Depression Inventory; SF-36=Short Form; WHO-CIDI=World Health Organization Composite International Diagnostic Interview; QI=Quality Improvement; CBT=Cognitive Behavioral Therapy; HAM-D=Hamilton Rating Scale for Depression; SIP=Sickness Impact Profile; MADRS=Montgomery Asberg Depression Rating Scale

Screening for Depression in Adults

**Appendix G Table 1. Evidence table of screening trials-KQ1 and KQ1a.**

| Study<br><br>USPSTF Quality | Study design<br>Point of randomization<br>Unit of randomization<br>Setting | Intervention and control conditions | Depressive disorders identified or targeted<br><br>% Currently treated for depression | Location<br><br>Population targeted | CONSORT numbers | Population characteristics<br><br>Baseline depression scores | Inclusion and exclusion criteria |
|---|---|---|---|---|---|---|---|
| **KQ1a trial** | | | | | | | |
| Rubenstein et al 2007[116]<br><br>Fair | Subgroup analysis of CCT<br><br>Clinics assigned to treatment group, participants enrolled after screening positive for one of 5 conditions<br><br>Primary Care | I: Structured phone assessment with case manager, then referrals as needed to (1) multidisciplinary geriatric assessment clinic; (2) home-based primary care program for homebound elders; (3) primary care provider; or (4) other specific services (e.g. mental health). Also health education and promotion, written summaries of recommendations, appointments, etc.. Called again after 1 month, then quarterly for 3 years.<br><br>C: Usual Care | Not specified, just positive depression screen<br><br>Curr tx: NR | Los Angeles, CA outpatient VA clinic<br><br>Age 65+ at risk for one or more of five common geriatric conditions (falls/balance problems, urinary incontinence, depression, memory loss, and functional impairment) | 2,646 mail questionnaires 2,382 returned questionnaires 1001 met criteria as high risk 792 enrolled in study<br><br>I=380<br>C=412<br><br>Among those with positive screen for depression:<br>I=95<br>C=111 | Mean age I=74.6 C=74.3<br><br>Female: I=3.7% C=2.7%<br>HS or beyond:<br>I=75.3%<br>C=76.5%<br><br>No statistical differences | Inclusion: age 65+, 1+ clinic visits in past 18 mos; screen positive for one of five conditions<br><br>Exclusion: live outside of 30 mile radius of clinic; already enrolled in geriatric services; living in a long-term care facility |

USPSTF=United States Preventive Services Task Force; AHRQ=Agency for Healthcare Research Quality; RCT=Randomized Control Trial; CES-D=Center for Epidemiologic Studies Depression Scale; I=Intervention; C=Control; MDD=Major Depressive Disorder; NR=Not Reported; AE=Adverse Events; PRIME-MD=Primary Care Evaluation of Mental Disorders; SES=Socio-Economic Status; GDS=Geriatric Depression Scale; GP=General Practitioner; GPSS=Geriatric Postal Screening Survey; PHQ-9=Patient Health Questionnaire; NS=Not Specified; BDI=Beck's Depression Inventory; SF-36=Short Form; WHO-CIDI=World Health Organization Composite International Diagnostic Interview; QI=Quality Improvement; CBT=Cognitive Behavioral Therapy; HAM-D=Hamilton Rating Scale for Depression; SIP=Sickness Impact Profile; MADRS=Montgomery Asberg Depression Rating Scale

Screening for Depression in Adults

**Appendix G Table 1. Evidence table of screening trials-KQ1 and KQ1a.**

| Study USPSTF Quality | Screening instrument Mode of administration Who administered and scored How results sent to clinician Diagnostic work-up | Follow-up | Outcomes Depression outcomes Other health outcomes Adverse events | Group selected for analysis Similarity to all randomized Similarity at baseline | Analysis | Results P values NS=p>0.05, *p< 0.05, **p<0.01 | Comments |
|---|---|---|---|---|---|---|
| **KQ1a trials** | | | | | | |
| Callahan et al 1994[112]<br><br>Fair | CES-D, HAM-D<br><br>In-person interview; CES-D performed during regularly scheduled visit; HAM-D at special visit within 2 wks of first visit<br><br>Research assistant | 1-month, 3-month, 6-month, 9-month | Depression: HAM-D, how assessed NR<br><br>Other: SIP, how assessed NR<br><br>AE: NR | Completers at 6 mo.<br><br>NR<br><br>Groups similar on sex, age, race, education, cognitive impairment, alcohol dependence, % depression diagnosis, % on medication associated with depression (e.g. narcotics), on antidepressants, mean # of diagnosis, HAM-D, SIP | Paired-comparison t-tests at 6 months | CES-D: all patients improved over 6 months**, no group differences in amount of improvement<br><br>HAM-D: % Responded I=13%; C=12% (NS)<br><br>SIP: All patients improved over 6 months (p-value NR), no group differences in amount of improvement | |
| Rubenstein et al 2007[116]<br><br>Fair | GPSS<br><br>Mail<br><br>Case manager completed more extensive work-up, referred to primary provider, specialty care as needed | 1-yr, 2-yr, 3-yr (only 1-yr results reported on subgroup screening positive for depression) | Depression: GDS<br><br>Other: None on subgroup screening positive for depression<br><br>AE: NR | Those screening positive for depression at baseline<br><br>NR<br><br>NR | Repeated measures ANOVA | Mean GDS Score: Baseline: I=8.7; C=5.0<br><br>1-yr: I=8.8; C=6.1 (Time*treatment interaction p=0.05) | |

USPSTF=United States Preventive Services Task Force; AHRQ=Agency for Healthcare Research Quality; RCT=Randomized Control Trial; CES-D=Center for Epidemiologic Studies Depression Scale; I=Intervention; C=Control; MDD=Major Depressive Disorder; NR=Not Reported; AE=Adverse Events; PRIME-MD=Primary Care Evaluation of Mental Disorders; SES=Socio-Economic Status; GDS=Geriatric Depression Scale; GP=General Practitioner; GPSS=Geriatric Postal Screening Survey; PHQ-9=Patient Health Questionnaire; NS=Not Specified; BDI=Beck's Depression Inventory; SF-36=Short Form; WHO-CIDI=World Health Organization Composite International Diagnostic Interview; QI=Quality Improvement; CBT=Cognitive Behavioral Therapy; HAM-D=Hamilton Rating Scale for Depression; SIP=Sickness Impact Profile; MADRS=Montgomery Asberg Depression Rating Scale

Screening for Depression in Adults

**Appendix G Table 2. Evidence table for depression treatment of the elderly**

| Study reference | Treatments addressed | Comparison conditions allowed | Databases searched and years | Inclusion/exclusion criteria | Unpublished data? Non-English language studies? | Consort numbers |
|---|---|---|---|---|---|---|
| Wilson et al 2000[121] | Antidepressants: TCAs, SSRI, MAOIs, and Atypical Antidepressants (Mirtazepine, Minaprine, Medifoxamine) | Placebo | CCDAN through 1999, includes: Medline: 1966-1999 PsycLIT: 1887-1999 EMBASE: 1982-1999 LILACS: 1982 -1999 CINAHL: 1982 -1999 SIGLE: through 1999 Psyndex (1977-1999) National Research Register (1999) Dissertation Abstracts International Biological Abstracts Cochrane Controlled Trials Register Cochrane Collaboration Depression Anxiety and Neurosis Controlled Trials Register Extensive hand-searching | Included: Placebo-controlled RCT; Depression by any criteria; described as elderly or all aged 55+ Excluded: Population of people with explicit diagnosis of other psychiatric disorder (dementia, alcoholism, bipolar); dose-response or testing combination; focus on maintenance treatment; literature review; trials reporting on electro convulsive therapy (ECT), prevalence studies, prescribing practice or risk factors. | Unpublished: dissertation abstracts Non-English: NR | CCDAN: 697 abstracts 108 articles reviewed 18 Included Hand-searches: 78 articles reviewed 5 Included |
| Cuijpers et al 2006[122] | "Psychological" treatments, including CBT, psychodynamic, reminiscence, problem-solving, behavioral activation, interpersonal therapy | Untreated control group or other treatment (psychological or not) | Medline, PsycINFO, Cochrane Controlled Trials Register, Dissertation abstracts Years: 1966-2005 | Included: RCTs; subjects aged 50 years or older with clinically relevant depressive symptoms Excluded: Studies in which the effects of the psychological treatment could not be distinguished from the total intervention | Unpublished: Yes Non-English: 0 | 2,355 abstracts reviewed 129 articles reviewed 25 trials included (in 34 articles) |

Appendix G Table 2. Evidence table for depression treatment of the elderly

| Study reference (Author Year/ RM #) | # included trials<br><br># directly relevant to current review (include control group, primary care setting, one of treatments in our scope)<br><br># participants total<br><br># participants in trials relevant to current review | Analyses used in this review | Qualitative results summary | Quantitative results summary | Quality rating |
|---|---|---|---|---|---|
| Wilson et al 2000[121] | Included trials: 23 trials total, 17 (n=1524 calc) with sufficient data for meta-analysis<br><br>Subset of MDD: 8 trials (n=1,120 calc)<br>Subset of community-dwelling: 7 trials (n=1,070 calc) | Overall analysis, community-dwelling subgroup analysis<br><br>Compare analysis of 4-week outcomes subgroup with overall results to see if overall results likely heavily influenced or different from longer follow-up studies. | TCAs, SSRIs, and MAOIs are effective in treatment of older community patients and inpatients. | Odds ratios for depression at outcome:<br>TCA vs Placebo: 0.32<br>SSRIs vs Placebo: 0.51<br>MAOIs vs Placebo: 0.17<br>Atypicals vs Placebo: 0.52<br>Community-dwelling: 0.47<br>MDD subset: 0.44<br>(all p<0.05)<br><br>Percent of depressed at follow-up:<br>TCA vs. Placebo: 51% vs. 75%<br>SSRI vs. Placebo: 72% vs. 83%<br>MAOI vs. Placebo: 59% vs. 90%<br>Community-dwelling:<br>  Drug 64% vs Placebo 79%<br>MDD subset:<br>  Drug 64% vs Placebo 80%<br>(all p<0.05) | Good |
| Cuijpers et al 2006[122] | Trials: 25 (n=1,937), 21 included in meta-analysis (N=NR) | Overall analysis; analysis limited to those with waiting list as control group. | Psychological interventions are effective in reducing depression in depressed elderly. | Odds ratio for remission: 2.63 (1.96, 3.47)<br><br>Effect side for symptom report (average of clinican and self-report): 0.72 (0.59, 0.85) | Good |

**Appendix G Table 2. Evidence table for depression treatment of the elderly**

| Study reference (Author Year/ RM #) | Treatments addressed | Comparison conditions allowed | Databases searched and years | Inclusion/exclusion criteria | Unpublished data? Non-English language studies? | Consort numbers |
|---|---|---|---|---|---|---|
| Pinquart et al, 2006[120] | Pharmacological: TCAs, SSRI, MAOIs, other newer agents (e.g., venlafaxine, mirtazapine)<br><br>Psychological: "rational" (e.g., cognitive and/or behavioral), "emotive" (e.g., supportive, dynamic, interpersonal) | Placebo, control without active agent (attention-placebo OK) | Medline, Cochrane Database, PsycINFO, PSYNDEX Years: through 2004 (personal communication) | Included: mean or median age ≥60; MDD, dysthymia, minor depression; intervention group compared with control group; depression or psychological well-being outcomes; sufficient data to calculate effect size<br><br>Excluded: studies of maintenance treatment, combination treatment, and collaborative care treatment | Unpublished: Yes Non-English: 8 | 120 potentially eligible trials<br><br>Exclusions:<br>non-depressed pts (15) duplicate datasets (6) age cut-off (3) maintenance treatment (3) inadequate control group (1) didn't separate pharmacotherapy and psychotherapy results (2) only reported responders (1) |

**Appendix G Table 2. Evidence table for depression treatment of the elderly**

| Study reference (Author Year/ RM #) | # included trials<br><br># directly relevant to current review (include control group, primary care setting, one of treatments in our scope)<br><br># participants total<br><br># participants in trials relevant to current review | Analyses used in this review | Qualitative results summary | Quantitative results summary | Quality rating |
|---|---|---|---|---|---|
| Pinquart et al, 2006[120] | Trials:<br>Total 89 trials (62 antidepressants, 32 psychotherapy (5 both))<br>Relevant trials: could not ascertain directly relevant<br>Subset focus on MDD: 31 trials<br><br>Participants: 5,328 participants<br>Relevant participants: could not ascertain directly relevant<br>MDD subset: NR | Overall<br>MDD-only subgroup | Pharmacotherapy and psychotherapy are effective in reducing depression in depressed elderly; psychotherapy may be more effective in treating dysthymia and minor depression than pharmacotherapy, but they appear equally effective for MDD. | Pharmacotherapy:<br>Self-reported depression<br>d (effect size) = -0.62<br>$p < 0.001$<br>Q (homogeneity) = 65.9<br>Clinician-rated depression<br>d (effect size) = -0.69<br>$p < 0.001$<br>Q (homogeneity) = 292.4<br><br>Psychotherapy:<br>Self-reported depression<br>d (effect size) = -0.83<br>$p < 0.001$<br>Q (homogeneity) = 99.5<br>Clinician-rated depression<br>d (effect size) = -1.09<br>$p < 0.001$<br>Q (homogeneity) = 52.5 | Good |

TCA-tricyclic antidepressant; SSRI-selective serotonin reuptake inhibitor; MAOI-monoamine oxidase inhibitor; RCT-randomized controlled trial; NR-not reported; CBT-cognitive behavioral therapy; calc-calculated; MDD-major depressive disorder.

**Appendix G Table 3. Suicide Related Events in MDD and Other Psychiatric Indications**[124,125]

| Indication | | Event | Test Drug | Placebo |
|---|---|---|---|---|
| **Major Depressive Disorder** | | Completed suicide | 4/22379 | 1/14873 |
| | | | 0.02% | 0.01% |
| | *Behaviors* | Suicide attempt and preparatory acts | 48/22379 | 31/14873 |
| | | | 0.21% | 0.21% |
| | | Suicidal ideation | 111/22379 | 91/14873 |
| | | | 0.50% | 0.61% |
| **Other Psychiatric Disorders** | | Completed suicide | 1/15061 | 1/10573 |
| | | | 0.01% | 0.01% |
| | *Behaviors* | Suicide attempt and preparatory acts | 24/15061 | 13/10573 |
| | | | 0.16% | 0.12% |
| | | Suicidal ideation | 52/15061 | 51/10573 |
| | | | 0.35% | 0.48% |
| **Combined** | | | | |
| All Psychiatric Indications (major depressive disorder, other depression disorders, other psychiatric disorders) | *Behaviors* | Completed suicide | 5/39799 | 2/27309 |
| | | | 0.01% | 0.01% |
| | | Suicide attempt and preparatory acts | 74/39799 | 47/27309 |
| | | | 0.19% | 0.17% |
| | | Suicidal ideation | 169/39799 | 148/27309 |
| | | | 0.42% | 0.54% |

Screening for Depression in Adults

**Appendix G Table 4. Evidence table of systematic evidence reviews and meta-analyses of suicide risk related to SSRIs.**

| | Data Included | Drugs | Trial and participants | Duration | Outcomes | Outcome category definitions | Quality concerns/Comments |
|---|---|---|---|---|---|---|---|
| FDA 2006 Safety group meta-analysis[124] Statistical group meta-analysis[125] Center for Drug Evaluation and Research Regulatory review Not quality rated Funding: FDA | Data provided to FDA through data requests to drug sponsors. Obtained data 9/2005 through 9/2006 | Test drug vs. placebo SSRI: Citalopram Escitalopram Fluoxetine Fluvoxamine Paroxetine Sertraline Other: Duloxetine Venlafaxine Bupropion Mirtazapine Nefazodone 63% of patients were enrolled in trials of SSRIs SSRI 30,301 Active control 6,066 Placebo 26,042 | 372 RCTs (162 for MDD) Total Patients: 99,839 Test drug: 52,960 Placebo: 35,904 Active control: 10,975 Test drug w/MDD: 22,379 Placebo w/MDD: 14,873 **Psychiatric indications** Mean Age (SD) Drug: 41.8 (14.28) Placebo: 42.0 (14.48) 18-24 yrs: 9.6% ≥ 65 yrs: 8.8% Female Drug: 61.2% Placebo: 60.8% Race White Drug: 85.8% Placebo: 85.9% African-American Drug: 5.4% Placebo: 5.4% Asian Drug: 3.2% Placebo: 3.6% Hispanic Drug: 3.6% Placebo: 3.6% | 0-84 weeks MDD 0-16 weeks Mean: MDD 7.5 wks Other depression 26.5 wks | **Results preferentially chosen from the statistical group report.** Suicide (Psychiatric indications) Drug: 5/39,799 persons (1.3/10,000) Placebo: 2/27309 persons (0.73/10,000) OR (calculated): 1.72 (0.28, 18.01) Suicides in **MDD** Drug: 4/22,379 persons (1.79/10,000) Placebo: 1/14,873 persons (0.67/10,000) OR (calculated): 2.66 (0.26, 130.94) Risk difference (calculated): 1.12 (-1.1, 3.3) Suicidal behavior (Psychiatric indications)* Drug: 79/39,729 persons (19.9/10,000) Placebo: 49/27,164 persons (18.0/10,000) OR 1.11 (0.77, 1.61) Suicidal behavior + Ideation (Psychiatric indications)* Drug: 248/39,729 persons (62.4/10,000) Placebo: 196/27,164 persons (72.2/10,000) OR (95% CI) 0.84 (0.69, 1.02) Suicidal behavior + Ideation (in **MDD**)* Drug: 163/22,309 persons (73.1/10,000) Placebo: 123/14,728 persons (83.5/10,000) OR (95% CI) 0.86 (0.67, 1.10) | Suicides: completed suicides Suicidal behaviors: suicides, attempts, acts toward imminent behavior Suicidality: suicidal behaviors, suicidal ideations | Meta-analyses are based on individual and trial level data. Suicide rates are strikingly lower than in all other reviews. Possible explanations relate to the way events were detected and categorized: 1) All potentially suicide related adverse events had to occur within the double-blind phase of the trials and were excluded if they occurred more than one day after discontinuation of drug or prior to randomization. Excluding events prior to randomization is desirable, particularly if events occurring during a placebo run-in are categorized as occurring during placebo treatment. However, given the high early discontinuation rates with these drugs, excluding events after discontinuation would involve undercounting which may have been differential since overall discontinuation rates are similar for drug and placebo, but reasons for discontinuation differ. 2) Manufacturers analyzed their own data to a pre-specified protocol and classified possibly-related suicidal events, without FDA independently checking the case-reports related to this classification. FDA report does not provide information on the number of events in the other 5 categories used (i.e., fatal events with insufficient information; self-injurious behavior with unknown intent; self-injurious behavior, non-suicidal intent; non-fatal events with insufficient information; other: accidents, psychiatric or medical adverse events). |

Appendix G Table 4. Evidence table of systematic evidence reviews and meta-analyses of suicide risk related to SSRIs.

| Data Included | Drugs | Trial and participants | Duration | Outcomes | Outcome category definitions | Quality concerns/Comments |
|---|---|---|---|---|---|---|
| | | | | *Numbers reported in figures are discrepant from tabular data.<br><br>**BY AGE GROUP**<br>***Young Adults 18-24 yrs***<br>Suicidal behavior (All psychiatric disorders)<br>Drug: 23/3810 persons (60.4/10,000)<br>Placebo: 8/2604 persons (30.7/10,000)<br>OR (95%CI) 2.31 (1.02, 5.64)<br>Suicidal behavior + Ideation (All psychiatric disorders)<br>Drug: 47/3810 persons (123.4/10,000)<br>Placebo: 21/2604 persons (80.6/10,000)<br>OR (95%CI) 1.55 (0.91, 2.70)<br><br>***Adults 25-64 yrs***<br>Suicidal behaviors (All psychiatric disorders)<br>OR 1.03 (0.68, 1.58) †<br><br>Suicidal behavior + Ideation (All psychiatric disorders)<br>OR 0.79 (0.64, 0.98) †<br><br>***Older Adults ≥ 65 yrs***<br>Suicidal behavior (All psychiatric disorders)<br>OR 0.06 (0.01, 0.58) †<br><br>Suicidal behavior + Ideation (All psychiatric disorders)<br>Drug: 12/3227 persons (37.1/10,000)<br>Placebo: 24/2397 persons (100.1/10,000)<br>OR (95%CI) 0.39 (0.18, 0.78)<br><br>†As reported in Stone 2006 | | |

**Appendix G Table 4. Evidence table of systematic evidence reviews and meta-analyses of suicide risk related to SSRIs.**

| | Data Included | Drugs | Trial and participants | Duration | Outcomes | Outcome category definitions | Quality concerns/Comments |
|---|---|---|---|---|---|---|---|
| Hammad 2006[137]<br><br>Center for Drug Evaluation and Research, FDA<br><br>Review of regulatory data<br><br>Not quality rated<br><br>Funding: FDA | Data provided to the FDA from manufacturers.<br><br>Includes parallel group RCTs from drug development programs that were performed through 2000.<br><br>Patients had MDD and other anxiety disorders. | Drug vs. placebo<br><br>SSRI:<br>Citalopram<br>Fluoxetine<br>Fluvoxamine<br>Paroxetine<br>Sertraline<br><br>Other-2nd generation:<br>Bupropion<br>Mirtazapine<br>Nefazodone<br>Venlafaxine<br><br>TCAs:<br>desipramine, amitriptyline, imipramine | 251 trials (207 for MDD)<br><br>Total patients: 51,000<br><br>*MDD trial:*<br>n =40,028<br>SSRIs:14,675<br>Other-2nd generation: 10,929<br>Placebo: 8,868<br>TCAs: 5,556<br><br>*Anxiety trials*<br>n=10,972 (44 trials)<br><br>Mean age: 36.6-38.7 yrs<br>Female: 51-58%<br>In/Outpatient settings: NR | 6-17 weeks | <u>Suicide-in MDD</u><br>SSRI: 6/14,675 persons (4.1/10,000)<br>Other-2nd generation: 9/10,929 persons (8.2/10,000)<br>SSRI/Other-2nd generation: 15/25604 persons (5.9/10,000)<br>TCAs: 4/5,286 persons (7.6/10,000)<br>Placebo: 2/8,868 persons (2.3/10,000)<br>OR SSRI vs. Placebo (calc): 1.81 (0.32, 18.37)<br>OR SSRI/Other 2nd generation vs. Placebo: (calc): 2.60 (0.60, 23.42)<br>Risk difference SSRI vs Placebo (calculated): 1.8 (-2.7, 6.3)<br><br><u>Suicides-in MDD</u><br>SSRI/Other-2nd generation: 15/3707 person-yrs (calc) (48/10,000)<br>Placebo: 2/1071 person-yrs (19/10,000)<br><br><u>Suicides-in Anxiety trials</u><br>SSRI: 1/1273 (7.9/10,000)<br>Other-2nd generation: 0/1273 (0/10,000)<br>TCAs: 0/319 (0/10,000)<br>Anxiolytics: 0/174 (0/10,000)<br>Placebo: 1/4327 (2.3/10,000)<br>OR SSRI vs Placebo (calculated): 3.40 (0.04, 267.02) | | Events attributed to randomized therapy if occurred during therapy or within one day of discontinuation- would not count suicides in anyone who was discontinued early due to adverse events or other issues.<br><br>Excluded suicides prior to randomization.<br><br><u>113 placebo-controlled trials (n=28,145)</u><br>5 suicides/3335 person-years (15.0/10,000)<br><br><u>94 active-only controlled trials (n=11,883)</u><br>16 suicides/1443 person-years (110.9/100,000) |

114

**Appendix G Table 4. Evidence table of systematic evidence reviews and meta-analyses of suicide risk related to SSRIs.**

| | Data Included | Drugs | Trial and participants | Duration | Outcomes | Outcome category definitions | Quality concerns/Comments |
|---|---|---|---|---|---|---|---|
| Gunnell 2005[138] BMJ<br><br>From MHRA report done for CSM Expert working group<br><br>Update in BMJ June 2006[139] Additional table provided by authors<br><br>Report of the CSM expert working group December 2004[105]<br><br>Regulatory review<br><br>Review of regulatory data<br><br>Not Quality Rated<br><br>Funding: None | Published and unpublished data provided to MHRA through 2003.<br><br>Additional paroxetine data was provided in December 2004 | SSRIs vs placebo<br><br>Citalopram (9 trials)<br>Escitalopram (34 trials)<br>Fluoxetine (135 trials)<br>Fluvoxamine (48 trials)<br>Paroxetine (57 trials)<br>Sertraline (156 trials) | 477 RCTs<br><br>Adults with **all indications** (MDD, plus others)<br><br>Suicide data: 342 trials with 40,826 patients. Excluded fluoxetine.<br><br>Non-fatal harms*: 52,503 patients 439 trials<br><br>Suicidal ideation*: 45,704 patients 439 trials<br><br>In-/Outpatient settings: NR Exclusion of suicidal patients: NR<br><br>Patient characteristics NR<br><br>*Updated numbers with those presented in BMJ update in 2006. | Follow-up duration not available for all trials.<br><br>Mean: 8-10 weeks | Suicide-excludes fluoxetine<br>SSRI: 9/23,804 persons (3.8/10,000)<br>Placebo: 7/17,022 persons (4.1/10,000)<br>OR (95% CI) 0.85 (0.20, 3.40)<br><br>Non-fatal harms*<br>(includes suicides for fluoxetine)<br>SSRI: 128/30,814 persons (41.5/10,000)<br>Placebo: 75/21,689 persons (34.6/10,000)<br>OR (95% CI) 1.21 (0.87, 1.83)<br><br>Suicidal ideation*<br>SSRI: 97/26,882 persons (36.1/10,000)<br>Placebo: 80/18,822 persons (42.5/10,000)<br>OR (95% CI) 0.80 (0.49, 1.30)<br><br>*Updated numbers with those presented in BMJ update in 2006. Paroxetine trials in original report, n=95; in update, n=57. | Suicide: Any fatal self harm, including intentional overdose and other overdose (except accidental overdose)<br><br>Self harm: any non-fatal self harm<br><br>Suicidal thoughts: any reports of suicidal thoughts or ideas. | Did not look at individual patient data.<br><br>Includes patients treated for conditions other than depression<br><br>No descriptive characteristics of patients in included trials or of trial inclusion/exclusion criteria.<br>Companies analyzed own data to a pre-specified protocol but also provide case reports to the MHRA for all reports of suicidal behavior. MHRA checked these for consistency and completeness, with further follow-up with the manufacturer as needed.<br><br>In young adults with four disorders other than MDD, there were proportionally slightly more events of both outcomes. |

Screening for Depression in Adults

**Appendix G Table 4. Evidence table of systematic evidence reviews and meta-analyses of suicide risk related to SSRIs.**

| Data Included | Drugs | Trial and participants | Duration | Outcomes | Outcome category definitions | Quality concerns/Comments |
|---|---|---|---|---|---|---|
| Data from GSK Briefing document 4/5/2006[131]<br><br>Not quality rated<br><br>Drug company review of internal data | Paroxetine only | Indications separated<br><br>57 RCTs-all indications<br><br>19 MDD trials<br><br>**In MDD trials**<br><br>*N:*<br>Paroxetine: 3455<br>Placebo: 1978<br><br>*Mean age:*<br>Paroxetine: 46 yrs<br>Placebo: 46.5 yrs<br><br>*% Female:*<br>Paroxetine: 59%<br>Placebo: 60% | | <u>Definitive suicide behavior-in</u> <u>**MDD**</u> (paroxetine only)<br>SSRI: 11/3455 persons (31.8/10,000)<br>Placebo: 1/1978 persons (5.1/10,000)<br>OR (95% CI) 6.7 (1.10, 149.40)<br>Risk difference (calculated) 26.8 (5.5, 48.0)<br><br>Number need to treat-to-harm 373 (208, 1818)<br><br><u>Definitive suicidal behavior or</u> <u>ideation-in</u> <u>**MDD**</u>-paroxetine only<br>SSRI: 31/3455 persons (89.7/10,000)<br>Placebo: 11/1978 persons (55.6/10,000)<br>OR (95% CI) 1.3 (0.70, 2.80)<br>Risk difference (calculated) 34.1 (-11.3, 79.5)<br><br>***Young adults 18-24 yrs***<br>Suicidal behavior with or without ideation-in MDD<br>Paroxetine: 5/230 persons (217/10,000)<br>Placebo: 0/104 persons (0/10.000)<br><br><u>Definitive suicidal behavior-in</u> <u>**MDD**</u><br>Paroxetine: 3/230 persons (130.4/10,000)<br>Placebo: 0/104 persons (0/10.000)<br><br><u>Definitive suicidal behavior-all</u> <u>indications</u><br>Paroxetine: 16/786 persons (203.5/10,000)<br>Placebo: 5/548 persons (91.2/10.000)<br>OR (calculated): | Definitive suicidal behavior: completed suicide; suicide attempt and preparatory acts.<br><br>**Events classified independently by Columbia University experts** | Noted that increase in suicidality was driven by younger patients. When stratified by ages, no increased suicidal behavior was seen in 25-64 and ≥ 65 yrs. Eight of 11 events of suicidal behavior in MDD patients occurred in patients aged 18-30 years.<br><br>All definitive suicidal behavior events in the paroxetine only dataset were attempts.<br><br>In psychiatric disorders other than MDD, there was no evidence of increased risk of suicidal behavior or ideation or of suicidal behavior alone in patients with all other indications or in subgroups of those with "all other depression" or "all other non-depression."<br><br>Used exact method for OR and CI (not Mantel-Haenszel with continuity corrected as earlier analyses). Mantel-Haenszel method substantially underestimated risk due to small and disproportionate events and imbalanced randomization in some trials.<br><br>10 of 11 patients with suicidal behavior had experienced improvement and 9 of 11 experienced a social stressor at time of attempt. |

Appendix G Table 4. Evidence table of systematic evidence reviews and meta-analyses of suicide risk related to SSRIs.

| Data Included | Drugs | Trial and participants | Duration | Outcomes | Outcome category definitions | Quality concerns/Comments |
|---|---|---|---|---|---|---|
| | | | | 2.26 (0.78, 7.92)<br><br>***Young adults ≤ 30 yrs***<br>Definitive suicidal behavior –in<br><u>MDD</u><br>Paroxetine: 8/612 persons<br>(130.7/10,000)<br>Placebo: 0/339 persons<br>(0/10.000)<br><br><u>Definitive suicidal behavior -all</u><br><u>indications</u><br>Paroxetine: 30/2037 persons<br>(147.3/10,000)<br>Placebo: 12/1422 persons<br>(84.4/10.000)<br>OR (calculated):<br>1.76 (0.87, 3.78) | | |

117

**Appendix G Table 4. Evidence table of systematic evidence reviews and meta-analyses of suicide risk related to SSRIs.**

| | Data Included | Drugs | Trial and participants | Duration | Outcomes | Outcome category definitions | Quality concerns/Comments |
|---|---|---|---|---|---|---|---|
| Fergusson 2005[130] BMJ<br><br>Systematic review<br><br>Fair quality<br><br>Funding: Canadian Institutes of Health Research | Published only<br><br>Searched: Medline 1967-June 2003; Cochrane Collaboration register of controlled trials<br><br>November 2004;<br><br>Pearled reference lists from 3 systematic reviews (2 Cochrane 2000; 1 UK evidence based guideline 1998) | SSRIs vs placebo or an active non-SSRI control including tricyclic antidepressants.<br><br>Search terms included: SSRI; Serotonin uptake inhibitors; Citalopram; Fluoxetine; Fluvoxamine; Paroxetine; Sertraline. | 702 RCTs reviewed 411 SSRI vs. Placebo 189 trials reporting fatal and non-fatal harms<br><br>10,557 SSRI patients 7856 Placebo<br><br>**All indications**<br><br>59% of trials in patients with diagnosis other than MDD.<br><br>91% of trials include > 50% female.<br><br>91% of trials included patients with mean age < 60 yrs. | 93% ≤6 months Mean: 10.8 wks | SSRIs vs Placebo 7 suicides; 29 non-fatal attempts<br><br>Suicides (fatal attempts) SSRI: 4/10,557 persons (3.8/10,000) Placebo: 3/7856 persons (4.0/10,000) OR (95% CI) 0.95 (0.24, 3.78)<br><br>Non-fatal attempts SSRI: 23/10,557 persons (21.8/10,000) Placebo: 6/7856 persons (7.6/10,000) OR (95% CI) 2.70 (1.22, 6.97)<br><br>Suicides and non-fatal attempts SSRI: 27/10,557 persons (25.6/10,000) Placebo: 9/7856 persons (11.5/10,000) OR (95% CI) 2.28 (1.14, 4.55) | Suicide attempts (primary): fatal and non-fatal acts of suicide<br><br>Fatal suicide attempts: self inflicted acts resulting in death indicated by primary study.<br><br>Non-fatal suicide attempts: overdose or suicide indicated by primary study. | Can't separate out fatalities for those with MDD only.<br><br>7% of trials > 6 months.<br><br>Adverse events may be limited by drop-outs from trials (46% of trials had drop-out rates > 25%).<br><br>Adverse events available in 189/411 trials of SSRI vs placebo and thus NOT for most patients. |

**Appendix G Table 4. Evidence table of systematic evidence reviews and meta-analyses of suicide risk related to SSRIs.**

| | Data Included | Drugs | Trial and participants | Duration | Outcomes | Outcome category definitions | Quality concerns/Comments |
|---|---|---|---|---|---|---|---|
| Khan 2003[126] Am J Psych<br><br>Review of regulatory data<br><br>Not quality rated<br><br>Funding: NR | Summary basis of approval reports obtained from the FDA for investigational SSRIs approved for use in the U.S. between January 1985 and January 2000. | SSRI (investigational at the time, subsequently FDA approved) vs other or placebo<br><br>SSRI:<br>Citalopram<br>Fluvoxamine<br>Fluoxetine<br>Paroxetine<br>Sertraline<br><br>Active control:<br>Nefazodone<br>Mirtazapine<br>Bupropion<br>Maprotiline<br>Trazolone<br>Mianserin<br>Dothiepin<br>Imipramine<br>Amitriptyline<br>Venlafaxine | Unspecified number of RCTs conducted in order to get approval for an investigational drug.<br><br>Total: 48,277<br>SSRI patients: 26,109<br>Placebo patients: 4895<br>Active controls: 17,273<br><br>Indications not stated.<br><br>Patient characteristics: NR | Not reported | <u>Annual suicide rate (all patients)</u> 0.66% (6.6/1000)<br><br><u>Suicides</u><br>SSRI: 38/26,109 persons<br>(14.6/10,000)<br>% (95% CI) 0.15 (0.10, 0.20)<br>Placebo: 5/4895 persons<br>(10.2/10,000)<br>% (95% CI) 0.10 (0.01, 0.19)<br>Active control: 34/17,273 persons<br>(19.7/10,000)<br>% (95% CI) 0.20 (0.09, 0.27)<br>OR SSRI vs Placebo (calculated):<br>1.43 (0.56, 4.64)<br>OR SSRI vs Active Control (calculated):<br>0.74 (0.45, 1.21)<br><br><u>Suicides by exposure years</u><br>SSRI: 17/2864 person-yr<br>(59.4/10,000)<br>% (95% CI) 0.59 (0.31, 0.87)<br>Placebo: 4/897 person-yr<br>(44.6/10,000)<br>% (95% CI) 0.45 (0.01, 0.89)<br>Active control: 31/4094 person-yrs<br>(75.7/10,000)<br>% (95% CI) 0.76 (0.49, 1.03) | Not reported | **Quality concern**: Suicides assigned to the drug the person was on at time of event-even if trial was primarily of another medication. Not clear how classified event if discontinued medication.<br><br>Information on trial setting or exclusion of high-risk subjects not given except that included patients lacked psychotic features and never had a hypomanic or manic episode. Other trial and participant information not given. Not clear if adults only. Active control combines second-generation investigational drugs with older, first-generation antidepressants. Likely included open-label and other longer time period studies (unlike 2006 FDA analyses).<br><br>Counted placebo-run in phase as placebo treatment, therefore events prior to randomization are counted.<br><br>**Comments**: Couldn't comparably ascertain suicide attempts.<br><br>Rates based on exposure years not available for fluoxetine.<br><br>Much higher rates than other studies-particularly for all indications-may be due to large number of active controls compared with placebos-indicates more severe patients. |

**Appendix G Table 4. Evidence table of systematic evidence reviews and meta-analyses of suicide risk related to SSRIs.**

| | Data Included | Drugs | Trial and participants | Duration | Outcomes | Outcome category definitions | Quality concerns/Comments |
|---|---|---|---|---|---|---|---|
| Storosum 2001[140] Am J Psych<br><br>Review of regulatory data<br><br>Not quality rated<br><br>Funding: NR | Published and unpublished studies of SSRIs submitted to The Medicines Evaluation Board of the Netherlands for approval for use from 1983-1997.<br><br>Also searched MEDLINE from 1990-1999 to locate additional long-term studies. | Double-blind, placebo-controlled trials.<br><br>Drugs being evaluated were not specified. | 77 short-term studies, 8 long-term studies, and 14 long-term studies from MEDLINE for the indication of MDD.<br><br>Studies of elderly patients and those with chronic depression excluded. Suicidal patients excluded in 64 trials; not reported in 10 studies.<br><br>Short-term: 12,246 patients Long-term: 1946 Long-term MEDLINE: NR<br><br>Shorter-term: 50 trials in outpatients; 10 in inpatients; 7 in and outpatient; 10 not reported. | Short-term studies: ≤ 8 wks (mean 5.8)<br><br>Long-term studies: >8 wks (mean 38.3, placebo-controlled phase varied from 24-52 wks); were withdrawal or extension studies for sustained responders<br><br>Long-term studies-MEDLINE: > 8 wks (placebo-controlled withdrawal phase ranged from 24 wks to 3 yrs) ; were withdrawal or extension studies for sustained responders | ***Short-term trials-likely MDD***<br>Suicide completion*<br>Drug: 7/7944 (8.8/10,000) persons<br>Placebo: 4/4302 (9.3/10,000) persons<br>OR (calculated): 0.95 (0.24, 4.42)<br>Suicide attempts*<br>Drug: 29/7944 (36.5/10,000) persons<br>Placebo: 17/4302 (39.5/10,000) persons<br>OR (calculated): 0.92 (0.49, 1.79)<br><br>***Long-term trials-likely MDD***<br>Suicide completion*<br>Drug: 2/1345 (14.9/10,000) persons<br>Placebo: 0/604 (0/10,000) persons<br>Suicide attempts*<br>Drug: 9/1345 (66.9/10,000) persons<br>Placebo: 4/604 (66.2/10,000) persons<br>OR (calculated): 1.01 (0.28, 4.51)<br><br>***Long-term MEDLINE-in MDD***<br>Suicide completion<br>Drug: 7/1440 (48.6/10,000) persons<br>Placebo: 1/889 (11.3/10,000) persons<br>OR (calculated): 4.34 (0.56, 195.72)<br>Suicide attempts<br>Drug: 9/1440 (62.5/10,000) persons<br>Placebo: 0/889 (0/10,000) persons<br><br>*Not significantly different | | Article states that most trials included patients who fulfilled DSM criteria for major depression, thus results are likely MDD patients in regulatory trials. |

**Appendix G Table 4. Evidence table of systematic evidence reviews and meta-analyses of suicide risk related to SSRIs.**
RCT-randomized controlled trial; MDD-major depressive disorder; SSRI-selective serotonin reuptake inhibitor; TCA-tricyclic antidepressant; NR-not reported; MHRA-Medicines and Healthcare Products Regulatory Agency; CSM-Committee on Safety of Medicines.

**Appendix G Table 5. Evidence table of cohort studies of suicide risk with SSRIs.**

| Study | Data Included | Drugs | Conditions | Time Period | Outcomes | Quality Issues/Comments |
|---|---|---|---|---|---|---|
| **USPSTF Quality** | | | | | | |
| Sondergard 2006[144] Int Clin Psychopharmacol<br><br>Funder: The Lundbeck Foundation<br><br>Fair-Poor Quality | Nationwide Danish cohort 1995-1999<br><br>Registry of all prescribed antidepressants<br><br>Registry of recorded suicides<br><br>**Taking antidepressant**<br>N: 438,625<br><br>**Not taking an antidepressant**<br>N:1,073,862 (is approximately a 25% random sample of the population) | **SSRIs:** citalopram, fluoxetine, fluvoxamine, paroxetine, sertraline<br><br>**Other:** mirtazapine, venlafaxine, negazodone, reboxetine<br><br>**Older:**<br>- TCAs (11)<br>- MAOIs:<br>  isocarboxazid<br>  moclobemide<br>- Tetracyclics:<br>  maprotiline<br>  mianserin | **Any indication:** 438,625<br><br>Any antidepressant dispensed-no consideration of previous treatment. Excluded those who purchased lithium.<br><br>Age: median 56 yrs<br><br>**SSRI:**<br>N: 338,558<br>% Female: 64<br><br>**Other:**<br>N: 58,596<br>% Female: 64<br><br>**Older:**<br>N: 153,540<br>% Female: 68 | **Followup:** up to 5 yrs | **Sample not taking antidepressants:**<br>Suicides:<br>671 persons; (6.2/10,000)<br>Suicide rates:<br>*Total:*<br>12.6 per 100,000 py;(1.26/10,000)<br>*Men:*<br>19.9 per 100,000 py; (1.99/10,000)<br>*Women:*<br>5.5 per 100,000 py;(0.55/10,000)<br><br>**Sample taking antidepressants**<br>Suicides:<br>1474 persons; (33.6/10,000)<br>Range of suicide rates (by medication type):<br>*Total:*<br>115.4-486.2 per 100,000 py (11.5-48.6 per 10,000 py)<br>*Men:*<br>202.2-463.6 per 100,000 py (20.2-46.4 per 10,000 py)<br>*Women:*<br>72.9-169.9 per 100,000 py (7.3-17.0 per 10,000 py) | **Quality Issues:**<br>Comparison sample not matched to cases- were "random sample of everyone else approximately 25%<br><br>Strong risk of confounding by indications in drug-specific rates due to not selecting new users only and treatment for all indications.<br><br>**Comments:** Suicide rates 2-3 times higher in men than women- whether treated or untreated<br><br>70% of suicides occurred during the 1st month. |

SSR-selective serotonin reuptake inhibitor; TCA- tricyclic antidepressant; MAOI- monoamine oxidase inhibitor; py-person years; F/U- follow-up; GP-general practitioner; RR-relative risk; AD-antidepressant.

**Appendix G Table 5. Evidence table of cohort studies of suicide risk with SSRIs.**

| Study | Data Included | Drugs | Conditions | Time Period | Outcomes | Quality Issues/Comments |
|---|---|---|---|---|---|---|
| **USPSTF Quality** | | | | | | |
| Simon 2006[129] Simon 2007[241] Am J Psych Funder: NIH Good Quality | Prepaid group practice in Washington and Idaho 1992-2003 Group Health Cooperative -Pharmacy records -Outpatient visits registration -Hospital discharge data -Mortality records from state and national death certificate data | **SSRIs:** citalopram, fluoxetine, fluvoxamine, paroxetine, sertraline, escitalopram **SNRI:** venlafaxine **Other:** buproprion, mirtazapine, nefazodone, trazodone **TCAs** | 65,103 patients with MDD, dysthymia or depressive disorder not otherwise specified. 82,285 episodes of antidepressant treatment 9,520 patients contributed 2 episodes 1,916 patients contributed >2 episodes Included if had not filled an antidepressant prescription in previous 180 days. Age: mean 44 yrs (5-105) % Female: 69.5 5107 episodes (6.2%) were in patients <18 yrs. | 6 months for all persons after antidepressant use initiated. Gathered data for 10.5 yr period. | **Suicides:** N: 31 persons (4.8/10,000) 4/10,000 treatment episodes *<18 yrs* 5.9/10,000 treatment episodes *≥18 yrs* 3.6/10,000 treatment episodes Male vs. Female: OR 6.6 95% CI (2.9, 14.7), but did not vary across age. **Attempts:** N: 76 persons (11.7/10,000) 9.3/10,000 treatment episodes Overall, 73 suicide attempts prior to prescription *<18 yrs* N: 314/100,000 persons 95% CI (160, 468) (31.4/10,000) *≥18 yrs* N: 78/100,000 persons 95%CI (58-98) (7.8/10,000) No difference by sex **Rate of entire covered population:** 1.7/10,000 | 10% Medicare 7% Medicaid Overall mortality in Group Health population 1992-2002 17/100,000 Risk of suicide deaths was not higher in the 1st month than subsequent months OR=1.2, 95%CI (0.5, 2.9). Deaths occur at about same rate over 6 months Risk of attempt was higher in the first month than subsequent 5 months OR 2.4 95% CI (1.6, 3.8). However, highest risk was in the month preceding treatment. |

SSR-selective serotonin reuptake inhibitor; TCA- tricyclic antidepressant; MAOI- monoamine oxidase inhibitor; py-person years; F/U- follow-up; GP-general practitioner; RR-relative risk; AD-antidepressant.

Screening for Depression in Adults

Appendix G Table 5. Evidence table of cohort studies of suicide risk with SSRIs.

| Study | Data Included | Drugs | Conditions | Time Period | Outcomes | Quality Issues/Comments |
|-------|---------------|-------|------------|-------------|----------|------------------------|
| **USPSTF Quality** | | | | | | |
| | Additional analysis of 70,368 patients from 1996-2005 | | | | **Relative odds (range) of suicide attempt from prescription date by sources of prescription** | |
| | | | | | ***>30 days prior***<br>Primary care: 0.47 (0.32, 0.69)<br>Psychiatrist: 0.69 (0.33, 1.45)<br>Psychotherapy: 0.40 (0.30, 0.54) | |
| | | | | | ***1-30 days prior***<br>Primary care: 1.90 (1.28, 2.81)<br>Psychiatrist: 3.57 (1.70, 7.48)<br>Psychotherapy: 3.35 (2.52, 4.45) | |
| | | | | | ***>30 days after***<br>Primary care: 0.16 (0.08, 0.30)<br>Psychiatrist: 0.56 (0.23, 1.37)<br>Psychotherapy: 0.23 (0.15, 0.36) | |
| | | | | | <u>Age > 25 yrs</u><br>***>30 days prior***<br>Primary care: 0.56 (0.33, 0.94)<br>Psychiatrist: 0.65 (0.21, 1.99)<br>Psychotherapy: 0.42 (0.27, 0.65) | |
| | | | | | ***1-30 days prior***<br>Primary care: 1.85 (1.06, 3.23)<br>Psychiatrist: 4.02 (1.34, 12.06)<br>Psychotherapy: 3.19 (2.11, 4.81) | |
| | | | | | ***>30 days after***<br>Primary care: 0.13 (0.05, 0.35)<br>Psychiatrist: 0.87 (0.26, 2.99)<br>Psychotherapy: 0.22 (0.11, 0.41) | |

SSR-selective serotonin reuptake inhibitor; TCA- tricyclic antidepressant; MAOI- monoamine oxidase inhibitor; py-person years; F/U- follow-up; GP-general practitioner; RR-relative risk; AD-antidepressant.

**Appendix G Table 5.   Evidence table of cohort studies of suicide risk with SSRIs.**

| Study | Data Included | Drugs | Conditions | Time Period | Outcomes | Quality Issues/Comments |
|---|---|---|---|---|---|---|
| **USPSTF Quality** | | | | | | |
| Martinez 2005[128]<br><br>BMJ<br><br>Funder: Medicines and Healthcare products Regulatory Agency<br><br>Good Quality | UK General Practice Research Database- contains clinical records from primary care<br><br>1995-2001 | SSRIs: citalopram, fluoxetine, fluvoxamine, paroxetine, sertraline<br><br>Other: flupenthixol, mirtazapine, reboxetine, tryptophan, venlafaxine<br><br>MAOIs: phenelzine, isocarboxazid, tranylcypromine, moclobemide<br><br>TCAs: amimtriptyline, amoxapine, clomipramine, dosulepin or dothiepin, doxepin, imipramine, lofepramine, nortriptyline, trimipramine, maprotiline, mianserin, trazodone. | N: 146,095 people with new antidepressant prescription (no antidepressants within last year)<br><br>Diagnosed with depression, bipolar disorder, or dysthymic disorder<br><br>Age: 10-90 yrs, 18% > 60 yrs<br>% Female: 65<br>% mild depression: 69 | 62,224 person-yrs<br><br>Observation in years-median (interquartile range):  0.66 (0.57-1.03) | **Suicides-All drugs**<br>69/146,095 persons (4.7/10,000)<br>*19-30 yrs:*<br>19/34,792 persons; (5.5/10,000)<br>*>30 yrs:*<br>50/106,016 persons; (4.7/10,000)<br><br>*Female:*<br>13/94,767 persons; (1.4/10,000)<br>*Male:*<br>56/51,328 persons; (10.9/10,000)<br><br>**Standardized incidence rate (age and sex):**<br>6.2 (95% CI 4.0 to 8.5) per 10,000 py<br>*Female:*<br>0.9 (0.1 to 1.8) per 10,000 py<br>*Male:*<br>11.7 (7.2 to 16.3) per 10,000 py<br>**Non-fatal self harm-All drugs**<br>1968/146,095 persons (134.7/10,000)<br>*19-30 yrs:*<br>747/34,792 persons; (214.7/10,000)<br>*>30 yrs:*<br>936/106,016 persons; (88.3/10,000)<br><br>*Female:*<br>1105/94,767 persons;(116.6/10,000)<br>*Male:*<br>863/51,328 persons; (168.1/10,000)<br><br>**Standardized incidence rate (age and sex):**<br>289.4 (95% CI 261.8 to 317.0) per 10,000 py.<br>No differences by sex. | Descriptive data clearly indicate differences in those treated with SSRIs vs. other s=especially TCAs (e.g., younger, increased history of self harm and referral to psychiatrists). Therefore drug-to-drug comparisons are confounded.<br><br>36/69 people (52%) were taking antidepressants at the time of death.<br><br>Self-harm events were primarily drug overdoses (81%). |

SSR-selective serotonin reuptake inhibitor; TCA- tricyclic antidepressant; MAOI- monoamine oxidase inhibitor; py-person years; F/U- follow-up; GP-general practitioner; RR-relative risk; AD-antidepressant.

Screening for Depression in Adults

125

**Appendix G Table 5. Evidence table of cohort studies of suicide risk with SSRIs.**

| Study | Data Included | Drugs | Conditions | Time Period | Outcomes | Quality Issues/Comments |
|-------|---------------|-------|------------|-------------|----------|-------------------------|
| **USPSTF Quality** | | | | | | |
| Jick 1995[127] BMJ Funder: Pharmaceutical companies, RW Johnson Pharmaceutical Research Institute Fair Quality | UK General Practice Research Database - primary care records 1988-1993 | SSRIs: fluoxetine TCAs: dothiepin, amitriptyline, clomipramine, imipramine, lofepramine, doxepin Tetracyclic: mianserin Other: trazodone, flupenthixol | N: 172,598 of all indications 1,198,303 prescriptions 67/143 had history of suicidal behavior or had been prescribed >1 antidepressant 112/143 had documentation of depressive illness | 6 mo after antidepressant prescribed 167,819 py | <u>Suicides</u> 143/172,598 persons (8.3/10,000) 8.5 (95% CI 7.2, 10.0) per 10,000 py | **Quality Issues:** Death ascertainment mostly limited to medical records. **Comments:** In nested case control analyses, men had 2.8 (95% CI 1.9, 4.0) greater risk of suicide. |
| Mackay 1999[147] Brit J of Gen Prac Mackay 1997[145] Pharm and Drug Safety Funder: Drug Safety Research Unit Fair-Poor Quality | UK Prescription Event Monitoring Database -includes data studies monitoring 6 newly released antidepressants 1989-1996. Surveys of GPs six months following the first prescription for each patient in immediate post-marketing period. Response rates 55-64%. | SSRIs: fluoxetine, sertraline, paroxetine Other: nefazodone, venlafaxine, moclobemide | N: 74,748 patients of all indications (>80% depression) Mean age: 45.5-50.1 Female: 62.1-69.8% | 6 mo | <u>Suicide and parasuicide-All drugs</u> 2.7-5.6 per 1000 patient months (324-672/10,000 py) | **Quality Issues:** Low survey response rate (55-64%) and possible differential reporting of those with or without the events. **Comments:** All analyses excluded patients treated for mania, hypermania, agitation, or anxiety. Report of mania: 1.2 per 1000 pt-months of treatment during 90 days. Any type of death-All drugs-6 mo. 1098/74,748 persons (146.9/10,000-calculated) <u>Most frequently reported events in 1st month of treatment, range across medications:</u> Nausea/vomiting 26.3-71.9 per 1000 pt-months Malaise 9.9-25.0 per |

SSR-selective serotonin reuptake inhibitor; TCA- tricyclic antidepressant; MAOI- monoamine oxidase inhibitor; py-person years; F/U- follow-up; GP-general practitioner; RR-relative risk; AD-antidepressant.

Screening for Depression in Adults

126

**Appendix G Table 5.   Evidence table of cohort studies of suicide risk with SSRIs.**

| Study | Data Included | Drugs | Conditions | Time Period | Outcomes | Quality Issues/Comments |
|---|---|---|---|---|---|---|
| **USPSTF Quality** | | | | | | |
| | | | | | | 100 pt months Headache 12.5-25.1 per 1000 pt-months. Dizziness 6.7-31.9 per 1000 pt-months Drowsiness 7.3-25.5 per 1000 pt-months |
| (Data specific to Mackay 1997[145] | Four studies from Prescription Monitoring Database 1987-1992 | SSRIs: fluvoxamine, fluoxetine, sertraline, paroxetine | N: 50,150 of all indications (>70% depression) Mean age: 48.6-51.0 Female: 67.5-70.1% | 6 mo | **Suicides** 110/50,150 persons; (21.9/10,000) | Same quality issues. |
| Gibbons 2007[146] Fair-to-Poor Quality | US Veteran's Administration National Patient Care Database and Pharmacy Benefits Management Database 2003-2004 | SSRIs (agents not specified); non-SSRI 2nd generation (bupropion, mirtazapine, nefazodone, venlafaxine); TCAs | N: 226,866 with depressive disorders or unipolar mood disorders in medical record in 2003 or 2004 and no indication of depression in 2000-2002. 59,432 *not* treated with antidepressant 114,475 treated with one class of antidepressants 52,959 treated with >1 class of antidepressants Mean age: 57.4 yrs (SD 14.8) Female: 8.4% | 6-24 months of follow-up | **Suicide attempts** 36.4/10,000, among those treated with SSRI alone or in combination with other antidepressants 33.5/10,000 among those not treated with an antidepressant | **Quality Issues**: Drug-to-drug comparison distorted due to confounding by indication; did not statistically control for indicators of severity and more patients with MDD treated with non-SSRIs than SSRIs. Examined subgroup of those taking only one type of antidepressant-not representative of any treatment practice. Therefore, most analyses exclude 52,959/167,434 (32%) of those treated as they used combinations of medications. **Comments**: Did not examine suicide deaths |

SSR-selective serotonin reuptake inhibitor; TCA- tricyclic antidepressant; MAOI- monoamine oxidase inhibitor; py-person years; F/U- follow-up; GP-general practitioner; RR-relative risk; AD-antidepressant.

Screening for Depression in Adults

Appendix G Table 6. Evidence table of studies of discontinuation of SSRIs.

| Study | Data Included | Drugs | Trials and Participants | Time Period/Follow-up | Outcomes | Comments | Quality |
|---|---|---|---|---|---|---|---|
| **Meta-analyses/Systematic Reviews of RCTs** | | | | | | | |
| Arroll 2005[72] <br><br> Systematic Review | Published articles through 2004 involving RCTs of SSRI or TCA vs placebo in adult **primary care patients**. Studies of primarily children or elderly were excluded. | Sertraline (2); Escitalopram (3); Citalopram (1) | 4 trials of SSRI vs placebo addressed discontinuation <br><br> 3 trials included only those with MDD; 1 had heterogenous depression diagnoses <br><br> N: 1149 participants <br><br> Sample characteristics NR | 6-24 weeks | **Discontinuation due to AE (4 studies)** <br> SSRI: 5.2% (30/576) <br> Placebo: 2.6% (15/573) <br> RR (Fixed; 95% CI): 2.01 (1.10-3.69) <br> P<0.02 | All 4 studies were commercially funded - receiver was not. <br><br> Sensitivity analyses found no difference for high quality vs low quality studies in primary analysis | Good |
| Mulrow 2000[95] <br><br> Williams 2000[75] <br><br> Meta-analysis | Published and unpublished RCTs measuring clinical outcomes for any of 32 newer antidepressants with another antidepressant, psychosocial intervention, or placebo in **primary care or general practice setting**. Searched 1980-Jan 1998; many databases and extensive hand-searching | Newer meds for treating depression: Fluoxetine, Fluvoxamine, Paroxetine, Sertraline, Citalopram, Indalpine, Tomoxetine, Litoxetine, Femoxetine, Venlafaxine, Milnacipran, Mirtazapine, Viloxazine, Reboxetin, Moclobemine, Medifoxamine, Brofaromine, Toloxatone, Nefazodone, Ritanserin, Gepirone, Ipsapirone, Tandospirone, Felsinoxan, Fengabine, Amisulpride, Sulpiride, Bupropion, Minaprine, St. John's Wort | 28 trials with 90% or more of patients related to primary care <br><br> N: 5940 <br> Mean age: 45 years <br> Female: 71% <br><br> Depressed adults <br><br> Other sample characteristics NR | Required > 6 weeks; most were 6-8 weeks (up to 24 weeks) | **Discontinuation due to AE** <br> SSRI (range): 6-11% <br> Placebo: 2% <br><br> (raw Ns NR) <br><br> **Overall drop-out rate** <br> SSRI: 16-29% | 27 trials from Europe; one from US. 20/28 funded by manufacturer; 8/28 not reported. Many trials used doses toward the lower range of standard dosages | Good - intent to treat analyses used throughout <br><br> Excluded patients with: <br> 1) Serious medical illnesses <br> 2) Cognitive impairment <br> 3) Alcohol abuse |

128

Screening for Depression in Adults

**Appendix G Table 6. Evidence table of studies of discontinuation of SSRIs.**

| Study | Data Included | Drugs | Trials and Participants | Time Period/Follow-up | Outcomes | Comments | Quality |
|---|---|---|---|---|---|---|---|
| Beasley 2000[91]<br><br>Meta-analysis by manufacturer | 25 US Investigative New Drug Trials (RCTs) comparing fluoxetine with placebo, TCAs, or both. Trials completed through 1998; likely includes unpublished data. | Fluoxetine ( 20-80 mg/d) | 25 trials of fluoxetine vs placebo<br><br>Patients with MDD<br><br>N: 4016<br><br>12-90 yrs old; mean 46 yrs<br><br>White: 92%<br>Female: 62%<br>Average run-in 1 wk<br>Depression severity and suicide history NR<br><br>Total patients in discontinuation trials: 2562<br>Fluoxetine: 160<br>Placebo: 952 | 5-12 weeks | **Discontinuation due to AE:**<br>*20-80 mg/d*<br>Fluoxetine: 13.7% (221/1610 calc)<br>Placebo: 6.0% (57/952 calc)<br>P< 0.001<br><br>*20 mg/d*<br>Fluoxetine: 9.0% (62/690 calc)<br>Placebo: 7.7% (44/568 calc)<br>P< 0.39<br><br>**Total Discontinuation:**<br>*20-80 mg/d*<br>Fluoxetine: 37.7% (607/1610 calc)<br>Placebo: 38.2% (364/952 calc)<br>P=0.211<br><br>*20 mg/d*<br>Fluoxetine: 29% (200/690 calc)<br>Placebo: 27.5% (156/568 calc)<br>P=0.832 | Researchers from Eli Lilly<br><br>Includes patients under age 18 - but what % age is not provided<br><br>Excluded patients:<br>1) Improved ≥ 20% in 1 week placebo run-in<br>2) History of substance abuse<br>3) Serious suicide risk<br>4) Psychosis, unstable medical condition<br><br>Adverse events done by blinded investigation | Fair - due to potential conflict of interest and from lack of quality assessment (assumes all Investigational New Drug Trials are well done) |

129

**Appendix G Table 6. Evidence table of studies of discontinuation of SSRIs.**

| Study | Data Included | Drugs | Trials and Participants | Time Period/Follow-up | Outcomes | Comments | Quality |
|---|---|---|---|---|---|---|---|
| Gartlehner 2007[92]<br><br>Comparative Effectiveness Review | High-quality meta-analyses, head-to-head double-blind RCTs, or controlled observational studies. Searched 1980-Feb 2006, included strategies for unpublished data. | 2nd generation antidepressants approved for us in the U.S.:<br><br>Buproprion, Citalopram, Duloxetine, Escitalopram, Fluoxetine, Fluvoxamine, Mirtazapine, Nefazodone, Paraxetine, Sertraline, Trazodone, Venlafaxine | MDD, dysthymia, or subsyndromal depression<br><br>**Discontinuation**<br>N, trials: NR<br>N, patients: NR<br><br>Sample characteristics NR | Minimum 6 wks for RCTs, 3 months for observational studies | **Discontinuation due to AE**<br>SSRIs: 8.1%<br>Buproprion: 6.7%<br>Duloxetine: 5.5%<br>Mirtazapine: 9.5%<br>Nefazodone: 15.0%<br>Trazodone: 7.0%<br>Venlafaxine: 11.5%<br><br>**Total Discontinuation:**<br>SSRIs: 20.8%<br>Buproprion: 14.1%<br>Duloxetine: 17.2%<br>Mirtazapine: 21.6%<br>Nefazodone: 23.6%<br>Trazodone: 20.7%<br>Venlafaxine: 24.8% | Did not review all placebo controlled RCTs for this as it was a Comparative effectiveness review.<br><br>Reporting does not allow data for discontinuation to be verified | Fair - due to reporting |
| Mottram 2005[94]<br><br>Cochrane comparative effectiveness review | RCTs comparing two or more antidepressants in treatment of depression in older (55+) adults. Searched through July 2003, may have included some unpublished data. | SSRIs: Paroxetine, fluoxetine, citalopram, fluvoxamine, sertraline;<br><br>Other 2nd Generation: buspirone, bupropion, milnacipan, venlafaxine, reboxetine; | 18 trials conducted in outpatient settings primarily in 1302 patients with MDD, dysthymia, unipolar depression, or non-specified depression<br><br>N: 554 SSRI recipients<br><br>Sample characteristics NR | 4-8 weeks | (raw Ns NR)<br><br>**Discontinuation due to AE**<br>SSRIs: 17.3% (96/554)<br>Other 2nd generation: 8.0% (60/748)<br><br>**Total Discontinuation:**<br>SSRIs: 27.4% (152/554)<br>Other 2nd generation: 36.0% (269/748) | | Good |

**Appendix G Table 6. Evidence table of studies of discontinuation of SSRIs.**

| Study | Data Included | Drugs | Trials and Participants | Time Period/Follow-up | Outcomes | Comments | Quality |
|-------|---------------|-------|-------------------------|-----------------------|----------|----------|---------|
| Anderson 2000[90] <br><br> Meta-analysis | Published RCTs comparing efficacy and/or tolerability of SSRIs and TCAs in treatment of depression in adults. Searched MEDLINE through May 1997 and cross-referenced with previous meta-analyses and reviews | SSRIs: Paroxetine, fluoxetine, citalopram, fluvoxamine, sertraline; | 95 RCTs <br><br> N: 10,839 <br><br> Patients with unipolar major depressive illness <br><br> Sample characteristics NR | Most 4–8 weeks | **Discontinuation due to AE** <br> SSRIs: 12.4% <br> Adults 65+ SSRI or TCA: 21.8% <br> Adults <65 SSRI or TCA: 14.7% <br><br> **Total Discontinuation:** <br> SSRIs: 27.0% <br> Adults 65+ SSRI or TCA: 36.5% <br> Adults<65 SSRI or TCA: 29.2% <br><br> Raw Ns – NR | Reported that total discontinuation and discontinuation due to adverse events in elderly were similar between TCAs and SSRIs | Good |
| MacGillivray 2003[93] <br><br> Meta-analysis | RCTs comparing SSRIs with TCA in **adult primary care patients**. Searched Cochrane Depression, Anxiety, and Neurosis group database through April 2002. Included efforts to identify unpublished literature. | SSRIs and TCAs (did not specify agents) | 8 RCTs <br><br> Mean age 40–45 yrs 75% female in most trials Mostly Caucasian <br><br> Predominantly adults in primary care with depressive disorder | NR | **Discontinuation due to AE** <br> SSRIs: 11.6% (164/1416) 95% CI (9.9%, 13.3%) <br><br> **Total Discontinuation:** <br> SSRIs: 20.7% (264/1275) | Primary results robust to excluding or including poorer quality trials | Fair - due to limited search strategy |

**Cohort Studies/Uncontrolled Treatment Trials**

| Study | Data Included | Drugs | Trials and Participants | Time Period/Follow-up | Outcomes | Comments | Quality |
|-------|---------------|-------|-------------------------|-----------------------|----------|----------|---------|
| Rush 2006[46] <br><br> STAR-D | Treatment discontinuation after each of four treatment phases, only those unsuccessfully treated in previous step move to subsequent step | **Step 1**: Citalopram <br> **Step 2**: Bupropion; Sertraline; Venlafaxine; Citalopram plus bupropion, buspirone, or cognitive therapy; or Cognitive therapy <br> **Step 3**: Nortriptyline, Mirtazapine, Lithium augmentation, T3 augmentation, Bupropion, or Venlafaxine <br> **Step 4**: Tranylcypromine or Venlafaxine XR+Mirtazapine | Non-psychotic major depressive disorder <br><br> At initial treatment step: <br> Mean age: 40.7 yrs <br> Female: 62.2% <br> White: 76.8% <br> Black: 16.8% <br> Hispanic: 11.9% <br><br> Depression severity and history of suicidality NR | Average 8.6 - 10.1 weeks for each step | **Discontinuation due to AE\*** <br> Step 1: 16.3% (599/3671) <br> Step 2: 19.5% (281/1439) <br> Step 3: 25.6% (100/390) <br> Step 4: 30.1% (37/123) <br><br> \*Discontinuation <4 wks or indicated intolerance as reason for exit from study | | Fair |

**Appendix G Table 6. Evidence table of studies of discontinuation of SSRIs.**

| Study | Data Included | Drugs | Trials and Participants | Time Period/Follow-up | Outcomes | Comments | Quality |
|-------|---------------|-------|-------------------------|----------------------|----------|----------|---------|
| Kroenke, 2001[96]<br><br>ARTIST | Open-label intention-to-treat trial or **depressed primary care patients** | Paroxetine, Fluoxetine, Sertraline | MDD, Dysthymia, Minor Depression<br><br>Mean age:<br>47.2 (Paroxetine)<br>47.1 (Fluoxetine)<br>44.1 (Sertraline)<br><br>% Female:<br>76% (Paroxetine)<br>86% (Fluoxetine)<br>75% (Sertraline)<br><br>% White:<br>85% (Paroxetine)<br>88% (Fluoxetine)<br>79% (Sertraline) | Follow-up at 1, 3, 6, and 9 months | **Discontinuation due to AE at 9 months:**<br>Paroxetine: 30% (56/189)<br>Fluoxetine: 23% (44/193)<br>Sertraline: 24% (46/191)<br><br>**Total Discontinuation, by drug at 9 months:**<br>Paroxetine: 45% (85/189)<br>Fluoxetine: 34% (66/193)<br>Sertraline: 41%* (77/191)<br>*41% reported, but calculates as 40% from raw Ns<br><br>**Total Discontinuation, all drugs:**<br>1 mo: 13%<br>3 mo: 23%<br>6 mo: 32%<br>9 mo: 40%<br>(raw Ns NR) | **Total discontinuation:** Stopped taking antidepressant or switched to another antidepressant<br><br>Community-based primary care network research | Fair |

RCT- randomized controlled trial; MDD- major depressive disorder; SSRI-selective serotonin reuptake inhibitor; TCA-tricyclic antidepressant; NR-not reported; RR-relative risk; AE-adverse events.

**Appendix G Table 7. Studies excluded from the review.**

| Reference | Reason for exclusion |
|---|---|
| Ackermann RT, Williams JW. Rational treatment choices for non-major depressions in primary care: an evidence-based review. J Gen Intern Med 2002; 17(4):293-301. | Exclusive focus on minor depression |
| Addis A, Koren G. Safety of fluoxetine during the first trimester of pregnancy: a meta-analytical review of epidemiological studies. Psychol Med 2000;30(1):89-94. | Focus on pregnancy-related screening |
| Adler DA, Bungay KM, Wilson IB, Pei Y, Supran S, Peckham E et al. The impact of a pharmacist intervention on 6-month outcomes in depressed primary care patients. General Hospital Psychiatry 2004;26(3):199-209. | Focus on treatment comparison, matching, or fine-tuning |
| Alexopoulos GS, Raue P, Arean P. Problem-solving therapy versus supportive therapy in geriatric major depression with executive dysfunction. American Journal of Geriatric Psychiatry 2003;11(1):46-52. | Not a general primary care population |
| Ali S, Milev R. Switch to Mania Upon Discontinuation of Antidepressants in Patients With Mood Disorders: A Review of the Literature. Canadian Journal of Psychiatry 2003;48(4):258-264. | Not one of included study designs for relevant key question |
| Allard P, Gram L, Timdahl K, Behnke K, Hanson M, Sogaard J. Efficacy and tolerability of venlafaxine in geriatric outpatients with major depression: a double-blind, randomised 6-month comparative trial with citalopram. Int J Geriatr Psychiatry 2004;19(12):1123-1130. | Not one of included study designs for relevant key question |
| Ames D. Depression and the elderly. In: Dawson A, Tylee A, editors. Depression: Social and exonomic timebomb. London: BMJ Publishing Group; BMA House;Tavistock Square, 2001: 49-62. | Not one of included study designs for relevant key question |
| Arean PA, Alvidrez J. Treating depressive disorders: who responds, who does not respond, and who do we need to study? J Fam Pract 2001; 50(6):E2. | Does not report included outcomes |
| Arean PA, Gum A, McCulloch CE, Bostrom A, Gallagher-Thompson D, Thompson L. Treatment of depression in low-income older adults. Psychology & Aging 2005;20(4):601-9. | Focus on treatment comparison, matching, or fine-tuning |
| Arean PA, Perri MG, Nezu AM, Schein RL, Christopher F, Joseph TX. Comparative effectiveness of social problem-solving therapy and reminiscence therapy as treatments for depression in older adults. J Consult Clin Psychol 1993; 61(6):1003-1010. | Not one of included study designs for relevant key question |
| Arthur AJ, Jagger C, Lindesay J, Matthews RJ. Evaluating a mental health assessment for older people with depressive symptoms in general practice: a randomised controlled trial. Br J Gen Pract 2002; 52(476):202-207. | Focus on treatment comparison, matching, or fine-tuning |
| Arya DK. Suicidality and the use of serotonin reuptake inhibitors. Aust.N.Z.J.Psychiatry 1995;29(3): 517-518. | Not one of included study designs for relevant key question |
| Aursnes I, Tvete IF, Gaasemyr J, Natvig B. Suicide attempts in clinical trials with paroxetine randomised against placebo. BMC Med 2005; 3:14. | Updated/covered by a more recent SER/MA |

| Reference | Reason for exclusion |
|---|---|
| Badamgarav E, Weingarten SR, Henning JM, Knight K, Hasselblad V, Gano A, Jr. et al. Effectiveness of disease management programs in depression: a systematic review. American Journal of Psychiatry 2003;160(12):2080 -90. | Not a screening intervention trial with usual care control group |
| Bains J, Birks JS, Dening TR. Antidepressants for treating depression in dementia. Cochrane Database of Systematic Reviews 2005;(3). | Not a general primary care population |
| Bak S, Tsiropoulos I, Kjaersgaard JO et al. Selective serotonin reuptake inhibitors and the risk of stroke: a population-based case-control study. *Stroke*. 2002;33:1465-1473. | Baseline groups not comparable on age, and outcomes is strongly related to age. |
| Baker R, Reddish S, Robertson N, Hearnshaw H, Jones B. Randomised controlled trial of tailored strategies to implement guidelines for the management of patients with depression in general practice. Br J Gen Pract 2001; 51(470):737-741. | Not a screening intervention trial with usual care control group |
| Ballesteros J, Callado LF. Effectiveness of pindolol plus serotonin uptake inhibitors in depression: a meta-analysis of early and late outcomes from randomised controlled trials. J Affect Disord 2004; 79(1-3):137-147. | Focus on treatment comparison, matching, or fine-tuning |
| Barak Y, Aizenberg D. Association between antidepressant prescribing and suicide in Israel. Int Clin Psychopharmacol 2006; 21(5):281-284. | Not one of included study designs for relevant key question |
| Barak Y, Olmer A, Aizenberg D. Antidepressants reduce the risk of suicide among elderly depressed patients. Neuropsychopharmacology 2006; 31(1):178-181. | Not a general primary care population |
| Barbui C, Hotopf M, Freemantle N, Boynton J, Churchill R, Eccles MP et al. Treatment discontinuation with selective serotonin reuptake inhibitors (SSRIs) versus tricyclic antidepressants (TCAs). Cochrane Database of Systematic Reviews 2005;(3). | Focus on treatment comparison, matching, or fine-tuning |
| Barbui C, Percudani M. Epidemiological impact of antidepressant and antipsychotic drugs on the general population. Current Opinion in Psychiatry 2006; 19(4):405-410. | Not one of included study designs for relevant key question |
| Barlow J, Coren E, Stewart-Brown S. Meta-analysis of the effectiveness of parenting programmes in improving maternal psychosocial health. Br J Gen Pract 2002; 52(476):223-233. | Not a screening intervention trial with usual care control group |
| Barlow J, Coren E, Stewart-Brown SSB. Parent-training programmes for improving maternal psychosocial health. Cochrane Database of Systematic Reviews 2005;(3). | Not a screening intervention trial with usual care control group |
| Barrett B, Byford S, Knapp M. Evidence of cost-effective treatments for depression: a systematic review. J Affect Disord 2005; 84(1):1-13. | Comparative-effectiveness |
| Barsevick AM, Sweeney C, Haney E, Chung E. A systematic qualitative analysis of psychoeducational interventions for depression in patients with cancer. Oncol Nurs Forum 2002; 29(1):73-84. | Not a general primary care population |

| Reference | Reason for exclusion |
|---|---|
| Bartels SJ, Coakley EH, Zubritsky C, Ware JH, Miles KM, Arean PA et al. Improving access to geriatric mental health services: A randomized trial comparing treatment engagement with integrated versus enhanced referral care for depression, anxiety, and at-risk alcohol use. Am J Psychiatry 2004; 161(8):1455-1462. | Focus on treatment comparison, matching, or fine-tuning |
| Bauer M, Dopfmer S. Lithium augmentation in treatment-resistant-depression: meta-analysis of placebo-controlled studies. J Clin Psychopharmacol 1999; 19(5):427-434. | Focus on treatment comparison, matching, or fine-tuning |
| Bech P. Meta-analysis of placebo-controlled trials with mirtazapine using the core items of the Hamilton Depression Scale as evidence of a pure antidepressive effect in the short-term treatment of major depression. Int J Neuropsychopharmacol 2001; 4(4):337-345. | Screen not used in clinical care |
| Berardi D, Menchetti M, Cevenini N, Scaini S, Versari M, De Ronchi D. Increased recognition of depression in primary care. Comparison between primary-care physician and ICD-10 diagnosis of depression. Psychotherapy & Psychosomatics 74(4):225-30, 2005. | Not a screening intervention trial with usual care control group |
| Beusterien KM, Buesching DP, Robison RN, Keats MM, Tomlinson JR, Cofran KW, Bailit HL, Adler DA, Bungay KM, Schrammel PN, Goss TF. Evaluation of an information exchange program for primary care patients with depression. Disease Management 2000; 3(1):1-9. | Focus on treatment comparison, matching, or fine-tuning |
| Beutler LE, Scogin F, Kirkish P, Schretlen D, Corbishley A, Hamblin D et al. Group cognitive therapy and alprazolam in the treatment of depression in older adults. J Consult Clin Psychol 1987; 55(4):550-556. | Not one of included study designs for relevant key question |
| Bezchlibnyk-Butler K, Aleksic I, Kennedy SH. Citalopram--a review of pharmacological and clinical effects. Journal of Psychiatry & Neuroscience 2000; 25(3):241-254. | Updated/covered by another more recent SER/MA |
| Bijl D, van Marwijk HW, de Haan M, van Tilburg W, Beekman AJ. Effectiveness of disease management programmes for recognition, diagnosis and treatment of depression in primary care. European Journal of General Practice 2004; 10(1):6-12. | Used as source document only |
| Bijl D, van Marwijk HWJ, Beekman ATF, de Haan M, van Tilburg W. A randomized controlled trial to improve the recognition, diagnosis and treatment of major depression in elderly people in general practice: Design, first results and feasibility of the West Friesland Study. Primary Care Psychiatry 2003; 8(4):135-140. | Does not report included outcomes |
| Blanchard MR WA. The effect of primary care nurse intervention upon older people screened as depressed. International Journal of Geriatric Psychiatry 1995;10(4):289-298. | Focus on treatment comparison, matching, or fine-tuning |
| Blanchard MR, Waterreus A, Mann AH. Can a brief intervention have a longer-term benefit? The case of the research nurse and depressed older people in the community. International Journal of Geriatric Psychiatry 1999; 14(9):733-8. | Focus on treatment comparison, matching, or fine-tuning |

| Reference | Reason for exclusion |
|---|---|
| Blier P, Tremblay P. Physiologic mechanisms underlying the antidepressant discontinuation syndrome. J Clin Psychiatry 2006; 67:Suppl-13. | Does not address included outcomes |
| Bohlmeijer E, Smit F, Cuijpers P. Effects of reminiscence and life review on late-life depression: a meta-analysis. Int J Geriatr Psychiatry 2003; 18(12):1088-1094. | Not one of included study designs for relevant key question |
| Bourin M. Use of paroxetine for the treatment of depression and anxiety disorders in the elderly: a review. Human psychopharmacology 2003; 18(3):185-190. | Updated/covered by another more recent SER/MA |
| Brambilla P, Cipriani A, Hotopf M, Barbui C. Side-effect profile of fluoxetine in comparison with other SSRIs, tricyclic and newer antidepressants: a meta-analysis of clinical trial data. Pharmacopsychiatry 38(2):69-77, 2005. | Focus on treatment comparison, matching, or fine-tuning |
| Brannan SK, Mallinckrodt CH, Brown EB, Wohlreich MM, Watkin JG, Schatzberg AF. Duloxetine 60 mg once-daily in the treatment of painful physical symptoms in patients with major depressive disorder. J Psychiatr Res 2005;(1):43-53. | Focus on non-elderly adults |
| Breggin PR. Recent U.S., Canadian and British regulatory agency actions concerning antidepressant-induced harm to self and others: A review and analysis. International Journal of Risk & Safety in Medicine 2004; 16(4):247-259. | Not one of included study designs for relevant key question |
| Breggin PR. Suicidality, violence and mania caused by selective serotonin reuptake inhibitors (SSRIs): A review and analysis. International Journal of Risk & Safety in Medicine 16(1), 31-49. 2003. | Not one of included study designs for relevant key question |
| Bruce ML, Ten Have TR, Reynolds CFI, Katz II, Schulberg HC, Mulsant BH et al. Reducing Suicidal Ideation and Depressive Symptoms in Depressed Older Primary Care Patients: A Randomized Controlled Trial. JAMA: Journal of the American Medical Association 2004; 291(9):1081-1091. | Not one of included interventions |
| Buchberger R, Wagner W. Fluvoxamine: safety profile in extensive post-marketing surveillance. Pharmacopsychiatry 2002; 35(3):101-108. | Updated/covered by another more recent SER/MA |
| Burke WJ. Escitalopram. Expert Opinion on Investigational Drugs 2002; 11(10):1477-1486. | Updated/covered by another more recent SER/MA |
| Burt VK, Wohlreich MM, Mallinckrodt CH, Detke MJ, Watkin JG, Stewart DE. Duloxetine for the treatment of major depressive disorder in women ages 40 to 55 years. Psychosomatics 2005; 46(4):345-354. | Not one of included study designs for relevant key question |
| Bush DE, Ziegelstein RC, Patel U, V, Thombs BD, Ford DE, Fauerbach JA et al. Post-myocardial infarction depression. Evidence Report: Technology Assessment (Summary) 2005; (123):1-8. | Not a general primary care population |
| Calil HM. Fluoxetine: A suitable long-term treatment. J.Clin.Psychiatry 2001;62(Suppl 22), 24-29. | Not one of included study designs for relevant key question |
| Callahan CM, Hendrie HC, Dittus RS, Brater DC, Hui SL, Tierney WM. Improving treatment of late life depression in primary care: a randomized clinical trial. J Am Geriatr Soc 1994; 42(8):839-846. | Does not report included outcomes |

| Reference | Reason for exclusion |
|---|---|
| Carroll BJ. Citalopram and the Curate's egg in geriatric depression. Am J Psychiatry 2005; 162(9):1762-1763. | Not one of included study designs for relevant key question |
| Casacalenda N, Perry JC, Looper K. Remission in major depressive disorder: a comparison of pharmacotherapy, psychotherapy, and control conditions. Am J Psychiatry 2002; 159(8):1354-1360. | Non-elderly treatment study |
| Cassano GB, Puca F, Scapicchio PL, Trabucchi M, Italian Study Group on Depression in Elderly Patients. Paroxetine and fluoxetine effects on mood and cognitive functions in depressed nondemented elderly patients. Journal of Clinical Psychiatry 2002;63(5):396-402. | Focus on treatment comparison, matching, or fine-tuning |
| Chisholm D, Sanderson K, Ayuso-Mateos JL, Saxena S. Reducing the global burden of depression: population-level analysis of intervention cost-effectiveness in 14 world regions. Br J Psychiatry 2004; 184:393-403. | Does not report included outcomes |
| Christensen KS, Toft T, Frostholm L, Ornbol E, Fink P, Olesen F. Screening for common mental disorders: who will benefit? Results from a randomised clinical trial. Fam Pract 2005; 22(4):428-434. | Missing both depression-specific screener and depression-specific outcome |
| Churchill R, Dewey M, Gretton V, Duggan C, Chilvers C, Lee A. Should general practitioners refer patients with major depression to counsellors: a review of current published evidence. Br J Gen Pract 1999; 49(446):738 | Years covered precede 1999 |
| Churchill R, Hunot V, Corney R, Knapp M, McGuire H, Tylee A et al. A systematic review of controlled trials of the effectiveness and cost-effectiveness of brief psychological treatments for depression. Health Technol Assess 2001; 5(35):1-173. | Updated/covered by another more recent SER/MA |
| Cipriani A, Brambilla P, Barbui C, Hotopf M. Fluoxetine versus other types of pharmacotherapy for depression. Cochrane Database of Systematic Reviews 2005;(3). | Focus on treatment comparison, matching, or fine-tuning |
| Cohen D, Hoeller K. Screening for depression: preventive medicine or telemarketing? Ethical Human Sciences & Services 5(1):3-6, 2003. | Not one of included study designs for relevant key question |
| Cohen JS. Avoiding adverse reactions. Effective lower-dose drug therapies for older patients. Geriatrics 2000;55(2):54-6, 59-60, 63-4. | Not one of included study designs for relevant key question |
| Cole MG, Elie LM, McCusker J, Bellavance F, Mansour A. Feasibility and effectiveness of treatments for post-stroke depression in elderly inpatients: systematic review. J Geriatr Psychiatry Neurol 2001; 14(1):37 | Not a general primary care population |
| Cole MG, McCusker J, Elie M, Dendukuri N, Latimer E, Belzile E. Systematic detection and multidisciplinary care of depression in older medical inpatients: a randomized trial. CMAJ Canadian Medical Association Journal 2006;174(1):38-44. | Focus on inpatient, residential treatment, psychiatric, or community settings |

| Reference | Reason for exclusion |
|---|---|
| Coleman CC, Cunningham LA, Foster VJ, Batey SR, Donahue RM, Houser TL et al. Sexual dysfunction associated with the treatment of depression: a placebo-controlled comparison of bupropion sustained release and sertraline treatment. Ann Clin Psychiatry 1999; 11(4):205-215. | Does not report included outcomes |
| Coleman CC, King BR, Bolden-Watson C, Book MJ, Segraves RT, Richard N et al. A placebo-controlled comparison of the effects on sexual functioning of bupropion sustained release and fluoxetine. Clin Ther 2001; 23(7):1040-1058. | Does not report included outcomes |
| Coleman EA, Grothaus LC, Sandhu N, Wagner EH. Chronic care clinics: a randomized controlled trial of a new model of primary care for frail older adults see comments. Journal of the American Geriatrics Society 1999; 47(7):775. | Not a general primary care population |
| Cookson J, Gilaberte I, Desaiah D, Kajdasz DK. Treatment benefits of duloxetine in major depressive disorder as assessed by number needed to treat. Int.Clin.Psychopharmacol. 2006;21(5), 267-273. | Focus on non-elderly adults |
| Corney R, Simpson S. Thirty-six month outcome data from a trial of counselling with chronically depressed patients in a general practice setting. Psychology and Psychotherapy: Theory, Research and Practice 2005; 78(1):127-138. | Focus on non-elderly adults |
| Cowen PJ, Ogilvie AD, Gama J. Efficacy, safety and tolerability of duloxetine 60 mg once daily in major depression. Current Medical Research & Opinion 2005; 21(3):345-356. | Focus on non-elderly adults |
| Coyne J, Palmer S, Sullivan P. Screening for Depression in Adults. Ann Intern Med 2003; 138(9):767-768. | Excluded study design |
| Croft H, Settle E Jr, Houser T, Batey SR, Donahue RM, Ascher JA. A placebo-controlled comparison of the antidepressant efficacy and effects on sexual functioning of sustained-release bupropion and sertraline. Clin Ther 1999; 21(4):643-658. | Does not repot included outcomes |
| Cuijpers P, van Lier PAC, van Straten A, Donker M. Examining differential effects of psychological treatment of depressive disorder: An application of trajectory analyses. Journal of Affective Disorders 2005; 89(1-3):137-146. | Focus on non-elderly adults |
| Cuijpers P. Psychological outreach programmes for the depressed elderly: a meta-analysis of effects and dropout. Int J Geriatr Psychiatry 1998; 13(1):41-48. | Intervention out of scope |
| De Lima MS, Hotoph M, Wessely S. The efficacy of drug treatments for dysthymia: a systematic review and meta-analysis. Psychol Med 1999; 29(6):1273-1289. | Exclusive focus on dysthymia |
| Delgado PL. Monoamine depletion studies: implications for antidepressant discontinuation syndrome. J Clin Psychiatry 2006; 67:Suppl-6. | Does not meet quality criteria |

| Reference | Reason for exclusion |
|---|---|
| Detke MJ, Wiltse CG, Mallinckrodt CH, McNamara RK, Demitrack MA, Bitter I. Duloxetine in the acute and long-term treatment of major depressive disorder: a placebo- and paroxetine-controlled trial. European neuropsychopharmacology : the journal of the European College of Neuropsychopharmacology 2004;(6):457-470. | Focus on non-elderly adults |
| Dew MA, Reynolds CF, Mulsant B, Frank E, Houck PR, Mazumdar S, Begley A, Kupfer DJ. Initial recovery patterns may predict which maintenance therapies for depression will keep older adults well. Journal of affective disorders 2006;65(2):155-66. | Focus on non-elderly adults |
| Dobscha SK, Corson K, Hickam DH, Perrin NA, Kraemer DF, Gerrity MS. Depression decision support in primary care: a cluster randomized trial. Ann Intern Med 2006; 145(7):477-487. | Not one of included study designs for relevant key question |
| Dobscha SK, Gerrity MS, Corson K, Bahr A, Cuilwik NM. Measuring adherence to depression treatment guidelines in a VA primary care clinic. General Hospital Psychiatry 2003;25(4):230-7. | Not a screening intervention trial with usual care control group |
| Donovan S, Clayton A, Beeharry M, Jones S, Kirk C, Waters K et al. Deliberate self-harm and antidepressant drugs. Investigation of a possible link. Br.J.Psychiatry 2000;(177): 551-556. | Not one of included study designs for relevant key question |
| Dowrick C. Does testing for depression influence diagnosis or management by general practitioners? Fam Pract. 1995;12:461-465 | Does not report included outcomes |
| Dwight-Johnson M, Unutzer J, Sherbourne C, Tang L, Wells KB. Can quality improvement programs for depression in primary care address patient preferences for treatment? Medical Care 2001;39(9):934-44. | Does not report included outcomes |
| Einarson TR. Evidence based review of escitalopram in treating major depressive disorder in primary care. Int Clin Psychopharmacol 2004; 19(5):305-310. | Non-elderly treatment study |
| Entsuah AR, Huang H, Thase ME. Response and remission rates in different subpopulations with major depressive disorder administered venlafaxine, selective serotonin reuptake inhibitors, or placebo. J Clin Psychiatry 2001; 62(11):869-877. | Sparse data on treatment vs. placebo in older adults |
| Ernst CL, Goldberg JF. Antisuicide properties of psychotropic drugs: a critical review. Harv Rev Psychiatry 2004; 12(1):14-41. | Did not report on an included intervention |
| Fabian TJ, Amico JA, Kroboth PD, Mulsant BH, Reynolds CF, III, Pollock BG. Paroxetine-induced hyponatremia in the elderly due to the syndrome of inappropriate secretion of antidiuretic hormone (SIADH). Journal of Geriatric Psychiatry & Neurology 2003; 16(3):160-164. | Not one of included study designs for relevant key question |
| Fahey T, Sullivan F, MacGillivray S. Screening for depression in primary care. Study analysis and conclusions are flawed. Bmj. 2003;326(7396):982 | Not one of included study designs for relevant key question |

| Reference | Reason for exclusion |
|---|---|
| Fava M, Amsterdam JD, Deltito JA, Salzman C, Schwaller M, Dunner DL. A double-blind study of paroxetine, fluoxetine, and placebo in outpatients with major depression. Ann Clin Psychiatry 1998; 10(4):145-150. | Not one of included study designs for relevant key question |
| Fava M, Hoog SL, Judge RA, Kopp JB, Nilsson ME, Gonzales JS. Acute efficacy of fluoxetine versus sertraline and paroxetine in major depressive disorder including effects of baseline insomnia. J Clin Psychopharmacol 2002; 22(2):137-147. | Non-elderly treatment study |
| Fava M, Judge R, Hoog SL, Nilsson ME, Koke SC. Fluoxetine versus sertraline and paroxetine in major depressive disorder: changes in weight with long-term treatment. J Clin Psychiatry 2000; 61(11):863-867. | Non-elderly treatment study |
| Fava M, Mallinckrodt CH, Detke MJ, Watkin JG, Wohlreich MM. The effect of duloxetine on painful physical symptoms in depressed patients: do improvements in these symptoms result in higher remission rates? J Clin Psychiatry 2004; 65(4):521-530. | Non-elderly treatment study |
| Fava M. Prospective studies of adverse events related to antidepressant discontinuation. J Clin Psychiatry 2006; 67:Suppl-21. | Not one of included study designs for relevant key question |
| Feighner JP, Gardner EA, Johnston JA, Batey SR, Khayrallah MA, Ascher JA et al. Double-blind comparison of bupropion and fluoxetine in depressed outpatients. J Clin Psychiatry 1991; 52(8):329-335. | Not one of included study designs for relevant key question |
| Ferguson JM, Shrivastava RK, Stahl SM, Hartford JT, Borian F, Ieni J et al. Reemergence of sexual dysfunction in patients with major depressive disorder: double-blind comparison of nefazodone and sertraline. Journal of Clinical Psychiatry 2001;62(1):24-9. | Not one of included study designs for relevant key question |
| Finkel SI, Richter EM, Clary CM. Comparative efficacy and safety of sertraline versus nortriptyline in major depression in patients 70 and older. International Psychogeriatrics 1999;11(1):85-99. | Comparative-effectiveness |
| Fishbain D. Evidence-based data on pain relief with antidepressants. Ann Med 2000; 32(5):305-316. | Non-elderly treatment study |
| Fraguas R, Jr., Gonsalves Henriques S Jr, De Lucia MS, Iosifescu DV, Schwartz FH, Rossi MP et al. The detection of depression in medical setting: A study with PRIME-MD. J Affect Disord 2006; 91(1):11-17. | Not a screening intervention trial with usual care control group |
| Frazer CJ, Christensen H, Griffiths KM. Effectiveness of treatments for depression in older people. Medical Journal of Australia 2005;182(12):627-32. | Does not meet quality criteria |
| Freudenstein U, Jagger C, Arthur A, Donner-Banzhoff N. Treatments for late life depression in primary care: a systematic review. Fam Pract 2001; 18(3):321-327. | Updated/covered by another more recent SER/MA |
| Friedman MA, Detweiler-Bedell JB, Leventhal HE, Horne R, Keitner G, Miller IW. Combined psychotherapy and pharmacotherapy for the treatment of major depressive disorder. Clinical Psychology: Science and Practice 2004; 11(1):47 | Non-elderly treatment study |

| Reference | Reason for exclusion |
|---|---|
| Furukawa TA, McGuire H, Barbui C. Meta-analysis of effects and side effects of low dosage tricyclic antidepressants in depression: systematic review. BMJ 2002; 325:991-999. | Non-elderly treatment study |
| Gartlehner G, Hansen RA, Carey TS, Lohr KN, Gaynes BN, Randolph LC. Discontinuation rates for selective serotonin reuptake inhibitors and other second-generation antidepressants in outpatients with major depressive disorder: A systematic review and meta-analysis. Int.Clin.Psychopharmacol. 2005;20(2), 59-69. | Updated/covered by another more recent SER/MA |
| Gastpar M, Singer A, Zeller K. Comparative efficacy and safety of a once-daily dosage of hypericum extract STW3-VI and citalopram in patients with moderate depression: A double-blind, randomised, multicentre, placebo-controlled study. Pharmacopsychiatry 2006;39(2), 66-75. | Non-elderly treatment study |
| Gatz M, Fiske A, Fox LS, Kaskie B, Kasl-Godley JE, McCallum TJ et al. Empirically validated psychological treatments for older adults. Journal of Mental Health and Aging 1998; 4(1):9-46. | Not one of included study designs for relevant key question |
| Geddes JR, Carney SM, Davies C, Furukawa TA, Kupfer DJ, Frank E et al. Relapse prevention with antidepressant drug treatment in depressive disorders: a systematic review. Lancet 2003; 361(9358):653-661. | Depression prevention or treatment maintenance interventions |
| German PS, Shapiro S, Skinner EA et al. Detection and management of mental health problems of older patients by primary care providers. JAMA. 1987;257:489-493. | Does not report included outcomes |
| Gerson S, Belin TR, Kaufman A, Mintz J, Jarvik L. Pharmacological and psychological treatments for depressed older patients: a meta-analysis and overview of recent findings. Harv Rev Psychiatry 1999; 7(1):1-28. | Not one of included study designs for relevant key question |
| Ghazi-Noori S, Chung TH, Deane KHO, Rickards H, Clarke CE. Therapies for Depression in Parkinson's Disease. Cochrane Database of Systematic Reviews 2005;(3). | Not a general primary care population |
| Gilbody S, House AO, Sheldon TA. Screening and case finding instruments for depression. Cochrane Database of Systematic Reviews 2005;(4):CD002792. | Not one of included study designs for relevant key question |
| Gilbody S, Whitty P, Grimshaw J, Thomas R. Educational and organisational interventions to improve the management of depression in primary care. JAMA 2003; 289(23):3145-3151. | Not one of included study designs for relevant key question |
| Gilbody SM, House AO, Sheldon TA. Routinely administered questionnaires for depression and anxiety: systematic review. BMJ 2001; 322(7283):406-409. | Not one of included study designs for relevant key question |
| Gill D, Hatcher S. A systematic review of the treatment of depression with antidepressant drugs in patients who also have a physical illness. J Psychosom Res 1999; 47(2):131-143. | Not a general primary care population |

| Reference | Reason for exclusion |
|---|---|
| Gill D, Hatcher S. Antidepressants for depression in medical illness. Cochrane Database of Systematic Reviews 2000;(4):CD001312. | Not a general primary care population |
| Gill D. Prescribing antidepressants in general practice: Systematic review of all pertinent trials is required to establish guidelines. BMJ March 15, 1997; 314(7083):826-827. | Not one of included study designs for relevant key question |
| Glassman AH, O'Connor CM, Califf RM, Swedberg K, Schwartz P, Bigger JT, Jr. et al. Sertraline treatment of major depression in patients with acute MI or unstable angina. JAMA 2002; 288(6):701-709. | Not a general primary care population |
| Gloaguen V, Cottraux J, Cucherat M, Blackburn IM. A meta-analysis of the effects of cognitive therapy in depressed patients. J Affect Disord 1998; 49(1):59 | Non-elderly treatment study |
| Goldberg D, Privett M, Ustun B, Simon G, Linden M. The effects of detection and treatment on the outcome of major depression in primary care: a naturalistic study in 15 cities. Br J Gen Pract 1998; 48(437):1840-1844. | Not a screening intervention trial with usual care control group |
| Goldberg D. The "NICE Guideline" on the treatment of depression. Epidemiol Psichiatr Soc 2006; 15(1):11-15. | Not one of included study designs for relevant key question |
| Goldberg HI, Wagner EH, Fihn SD, Martin DP, Horowitz CR, Christensen DB et al. A randomized controlled trial of CQI teams and academic detailing: can they alter compliance with guidelines? Joint Commission Journal on Quality Improvement 1998;24(3):130-42. | Not a general primary care population |
| Goldstein DJ LY. Duloxetine in the treatment of depression: a double-blind placebo-controlled comparison with paroxetine. J Clin Psychopharmacol 2004;(4):389-399. | Non-elderly treatment study |
| Grotzinger KM CB. Clinical outcomes after depression: improvement in clinical and economic outcomes after implementing a disease management program for patients with depression. 51st Institute on Psychiatric Services; 1999; 1999 October 25th-November 2nd; New Orleans, LA, USA 1999.:-November. | Not a general primary care population |
| Grunebaum MF, Ellis SP, Li S, Oquendo MA, Mann JJ. Antidepressants and suicide risk in the United States, 1985-1999. J Clin Psychiatry 2004; 65(11):1456-1462. | Not one of included study designs for relevant key question |
| Gunnell D, Ashby D. Antidepressants and suicide: what is the balance of benefit and harm. BMJ 2004; 329(7456):34-38. | Not one of included study designs for relevant key question |
| Guthrie E K. Randomised controlled trial of brief psychological intervention after deliberate self poisoning. BMJ (Clinical research ed ) 2001;323(7305):135-8. | Not a primary care population |
| Haby MM, Donnelly M, Corry J, Vos T. Cognitive behavioural therapy for depression, panic disorder and generalized anxiety disorder: a meta-regression of factors that may predict outcome. Australian & New Zealand Journal of Psychiatry 2006;40(1):9-19. | Non-elderly treatment study |

| Reference | Reason for exclusion |
|---|---|
| Hackett ML, Anderson CS, House AO. Management of depression after stroke: a systematic review of pharmacological therapies. Stroke 2005;36(5):1098-103. | Not a general primary care population |
| Hall WD, Lucke J. How have the selective serotonin reuptake inhibitor antidepressants affected suicide mortality? Australian & New Zealand Journal of Psychiatry 2006; 40(11-12):941-950. | Does not meet quality criteria |
| Hansen RA, Gartlehner G, Lohr KN, Gaynes BN, Carey TS. Efficacy and safety of second-generation antidepressants in the treatment of major depressive disorder. Ann Intern Med 2005; 143(6):415-426. | Focus on treatment comparison, matching, or fine-tuning |
| Hayes D. Recent developments in antidepressant therapy in special populations. Am J Manag Care 2004; 10(6:Suppl):Suppl-85. | Not a treatment outcomes study |
| Healey D. Lines of evidence on the risk of suicide with selective serotonin reuptake inhibitors: Reply. Psychother.Psychosom. 2003;72(6), 359-360. | Not one of included study designs for relevant key question |
| Healy D, Whitaker C. Antidepressants and suicide: risk-benefit conundrums. J Psychiatry Neurosci 2003; 28(5):331-337. | Not one of included study designs for relevant key question |
| Healy D. Lines of evidence on the risks of suicide with selective serotonin reuptake inhibitors. Psychother Psychosom 2003; 72(2):71-79. | Not one of included study designs for relevant key question |
| Henkel V, Mergl R, Coyne JC, Kohnen R, Moller HJ, Hegerl U. Screening for depression in primary care: will one or two items suffice? Eur Arch Psychiatry Clin Neurosci. 2004;254:215-223. | Does not report included outcomes |
| Hensley PL, Nadiga D, Uhlenhuth EH. Long-term effectiveness of cognitive therapy in major depressive disorder. Depress Anxiety 2004; 20(1):1-7. | Non-elderly treatment study |
| Hickie IB, Davenport TA, Ricci CS. Screening for depression in general practice and related medical settings. Med J Aust 2002; 177 Suppl:S111-S116. | Not one of included study designs for relevant key question |
| Hicks JA, Argyropoulos SV, Rich AS, Nash JR, Bell CJ, Edwards C et al. Randomised controlled study of sleep after nefazodone or paroxetine treatment in out-patients with depression. Br J Psychiatry 2002; 180:528-535. | Non-elderly treatment study |
| Himei A, Okamura T. Discontinuation syndrome associated with paroxetine in depressed patients: a retrospective analysis of factors involved in the occurrence of the syndrome. CNS Drugs 2006; 20(8):665-672. | Does not report included outcomes |
| Hippisley-Cox J, Pringle M, Hammersley V, Crown N, Wynn A, Meal A et al. Antidepressants as risk factor for ischaemic heart disease: case-control study in primary care. BMJ 2001; 323(7314):666-669. | Does not meet quality criteria |
| Hoeper EW, Nycz GR, Kessler LG, Burke JD, Jr., Pierce WE. The usefulness of screening for mental illness. Lancet. 1984;1:33-3 | Does not report included outcomes |

| Reference | Reason for exclusion |
|---|---|
| Hsieh HF, Wang JJ. Effect of reminiscence therapy on depression in older adults: a systematic review. Int J Nurs Stud 2003; 40(4):335 | Not one of included study designs for relevant key question |
| Hudson JI, Wohlreich MM, Kajdasz DK, Mallinckrodt CH, Watkin JG, Martynov OV. Safety and tolerability of duloxetine in the treatment of major depressive disorder: analysis of pooled data from eight placebo-controlled clinical trials. Human psychopharmacology 2005; 20(5):327-341. | Updated/covered by another more recent SER/MA |
| Huibers MJH, Beurskens AJHM, Bleijenberg G, van Schayck CP. The effectiveness of psychosocial interventions delivered by general practitioners. Cochrane Database of Systematic Reviews 2005;(3):223. | Non-elderly treatment study |
| Hunkeler EM, Katon W, Tang L, Williams JW, Jr., Kroenke K, Lin EH et al. Long term outcomes from the IMPACT randomised trial for depressed elderly patients in primary care. BMJ 2006; 332(7536):259-263. | Intervention out of scope |
| Hunziker ME, Suehs BT, Bettinger TL, Crismon ML. Duloxetine hydrochloride: a new dual-acting medication for the treatment of major depressive disorder. Clin Ther 2005; 27(8):1126-1143. | Does not address included adverse effects |
| Isacsson G, Holmgren P, Ahlner J. Selective serotonin reuptake inhibitor antidepressants and the risk of suicide: a controlled forensic database study of 14,857 suicides. Acta Psychiatr Scand 2005; 111(4):286-290. | Excluded for quality; high likelihood of confounding by indication. |
| Jarrett RB, Basco MR, Risser R, Ramanan J, Marwill M, Kraft D et al. Is there a role for continuation phase cognitive therapy for depressed outpatients? Journal of Consulting & Clinical Psychology 1998;66(6):1036 -40. | Non-elderly treatment study |
| Jarvik LF, Mintz J, Steuer J, Gerner R. Treating geriatric depression: a 26-week interim analysis. J Am Geriatr Soc 1982; 30(11):713-717. | Not one of included study designs for relevant key question |
| Jimenez-Jimenez FJ, Molina JA. Extrapyramidal symptoms associated with selective serotonin reuptake inhibitors: Epidemiology, mechanisms and management. CNS Drugs 2000;14(5), 367-379. | Not one of included study designs for relevant key question |
| Johnstone A, Goldberg D. Psychiatric screening in general practice. A controlled trial. Lancet. 1976;1:605-608. | Missing both depression-specific screener and depression-specific outcome |
| Juurlink DN, Mamdani MM, Kopp A, Redelmeier DA. The risk of suicide with selective serotonin reuptake inhibitors in the elderly. Am J Psychiatry 2006; 163(5):813-821. | Not one of included study designs for relevant key question |
| Karel MJ, Hinrichsen G. Treatment of depression in late life: psychotherapeutic interventions. Clin Psychol Rev 2000; 20(6):707-729. | Used as source document only |
| Kasper S, de SH, Friis AH. Escitalopram in the treatment of depressed elderly patients. Am J Geriatr Psychiatry 2005; 13(10):884-891. | Not one of included study designs for relevant key question |

| Reference | Reason for exclusion |
|---|---|
| Katon W, Von Korff M, Lin E, Simon G, Walker E, Unutzer J et al. Stepped collaborative care for primary care patients with persistent symptoms of depression: a randomized trial. Arch Gen Psychiatry 1999; 56(12):1109-1115. | Not a general primary care population |
| Katona C, Livingston G. How well do antidepressants work in older people: a systematic review of number needed to treat. J Affect Disord 2002; 69(1-3):47 | Updated/covered by another more recent SER/MA |
| Katzelnick DJ, Simon GE, Pearson SD, Manning WG, Helstad CP, HH et al. Randomized trial of a depression management program in high utilizers of medical care. Archives of Family Medicine 2000;9(4):345-51. | Not a general primary care population |
| Katzelnick DJ, Simon GE, Pearson SD, Manning WG, Helstad CP, Henks, HJ. Clinical outcomes care study. 152nd Annual Meeting of the American Psychiatric Association; Washington DC, USA; 1999. | Not a general primary care population |
| Kaye JL. Target complaints as a measure of outcome in psychotherapy with the depressed elderly. Dissertation Abstracts International: Section B: The Sciences and Engineering 2001; 62(5-B):2488. | Focus on treatment comparison, matching, or fine-tuning |
| Keller M. Lack of efficacy of the substance p (neurokinin1 receptor) antagonist aprepitant in the treatment of major depressive disorder. Biol Psychiatry 2006;(3):216-223. | Non-elderly treatment study |
| Kendrick T, Stevens L, Bryant A, Goddard J, Stevens A, Raftery J et al. Hampshire depression project: changes in the process of care and cost consequences. Br J Gen Pract 2001; 51(472):911-913. | Not a screening intervention trial with usual care control group |
| Kennedy GJ. New drugs for old folks: the evidence-based argument for newer antidepressants. J Am Geriatr Soc 2001; 49(2):227-228. | Focus on treatment comparison, matching or fine-tuning |
| Kessler D, Bennewith O, Lewis G, Sharp D. Detection of depression and anxiety in primary care: follow up study. BMJ 2002;325(7371):1016-7. | Not one of included study designs for relevant key question |
| Kessler D, Lloyd K, Lewis G, Gray DP. Cross sectional study of symptom attribution and recognition of depression and anxiety in primary care. BMJ 1999; 318(7181):436-439. | Does not meet inclusion criteria |
| Khan A, Brodhead AE, Schwartz KA, Kolts RL, Brown WA. Sex differences in antidepressant response in recent antidepressant clinical trials. J Clin Psychopharmacol 2005; 25(4):318-324. | Non-elderly treatment study |
| Khan A, Warner HA, Brown WA. Symptom reduction and suicide risk in patients treated with placebo in antidepressant clinical trials: an analysis of the Food and Drug Administration database. Arch Gen Psychiatry 2000; 57(4):311-317. | Updated/covered by another more recent SER/MA |
| Khan A. Severity of depressive symptoms and response to antidepressants and placebo in antidepressant trials. J Psychiatr Res 2005;39(2):145-150. | Non-elderly treatment study |

| Reference | Reason for exclusion |
|---|---|
| Kiev A, Feiger A. A double-blind comparison of fluvoxamine and paroxetine in the treatment of depressed outpatients. J Clin Psychiatry 1997; 58(4):146-152. | Comparative-effectiveness |
| Kirsch I, Scoboria A. Apples, oranges, and placebos: heterogeneity in a meta-analysis of placebo effects. Advances in Mind-Body Medicine 2004; 17(4):307-9; discussion 312-8. | Does not report included outcomes |
| Klausner EJ, Snyder CR, Cheavens J. A hope-based group treatment for depressed older adult outpatients. 2000. | Not a general primary care population |
| Klein DN, Santiago NJ, Vivian D, Blalock JA, Kocsis JH, Markowitz JC et al. Cognitive-behavioral analysis system of psychotherapy as a maintenance treatment for chronic depression. Journal of Consulting & Clinical Psychology 2004;72(4):681-8. | Non-elderly treatment study |
| Koren G, Matsui D, Einarson A, Knoppert D, Steiner M. Is maternal use of selective serotonin reuptake inhibitors in the third trimester of pregnancy harmful to neonates? CMAJ 2005; 172(11):1457-1459. | Focus on pregnancy-related screening |
| Krampen G. Long-term evaluation of the effectiveness of additional autogenic training in the psychotherapy of depressive disorders. European Psychologist 1999; 4(1):11-18. | Non-elderly treatment study |
| Krishnan KR, Doraiswamy PM, Clary CM. Clinical and treatment response characteristics of late-life depression associated with vascular disease: a pooled analysis of two multicenter trials with sertraline. Prog Neuropsychopharmacol Biol Psychiatry 2001; 25(2):347-361. | Not a general primary care population |
| Kurdyak PA, Juurlink DN, Kopp A, Herrmann N, Mamdani MM. Antidepressants, warfarin, and the risk of hemorrhage. J Clin Psychopharmacol. 2005;25:561-564. | Not a primary care population |
| Lane DA, Chong AY, Lip GYH. Psychological interventions for depression in heart failure. Cochrane Database of Systematic Reviews 2005;(3). | Not a general primary care population |
| Lapierre YD. Suicidality with selective serotonin reuptake inhibitors: Valid claim?. Journal of Psychiatry & Neuroscience 2003; 28(5):340-347. | Not one of included study designs for relevant key question |
| Lejoyeux M, Ades J. Antidepressant discontinuation: a review of the literature. J Clin Psychiatry 1997; 58:Suppl-5. | Not one of included study designs for relevant key question |
| Lenze EJ, Dew MA, Mazumdar S, Begley AE, Cornes C, Miller MD et al. Combined pharmacotherapy and psychotherapy as maintenance treatment for late-life depression: effects on social adjustment. American Journal of Psychiatry 2002;159(3):466-8. | Depression prevention or treatment maintenance interventions |
| Lepola UM LH. Escitalopram (10-20 mg/day) is effective and well tolerated in a placebo-controlled study in depression in primary care. Int Clin Psychopharmacol 2003;(4):211-217. | Non-elderly treatment study |

| Reference | Reason for exclusion |
|---|---|
| Levkovitz Y, Shahar G, Native G, Hirsfeld E, Treves I, Krieger I et al. Group interpersonal psychotherapy for patients with major depression disorder - pilot study. Journal of Affective Disorders 2000;60(3):191-5. | Non-elderly treatment study |
| Lewis G, Sharp D, Bartholomew J, Pelosi AJ. Computerized assessment of common mental disorders in primary care: effect on clinical outcome. Fam Pract. 1996;13:120-126. | Missing both depression-specific screener and depression-specific outcomes |
| Lexchin J, Bero LA, Djulbegovic B, Clark O. Pharmaceutical industry sponsorship and research outcome and quality: systematic review. BMJ 2003; 326(7400):1167-1170. | Does not report included outcomes |
| Lima MS, Hotopf M. Pharmacotherapy for dysthymia. Cochrane Database of Systematic Reviews 2005;(3). | Exclusive focus on dysthymia |
| Lima MS, Moncrieff J. Drugs versus placebo for dysthymia. Cochrane Database of Systematic Reviews 2005;(3). | Exclusive focus on dysthymia |
| Lin EH, VonKorff M, Russo J, Katon W, Simon GE, Unutzer J et al. Can depression treatment in primary care reduce disability? A stepped care approach. Arch Fam Med 2000; 9(10):1052-1058. | Not a general primary care population |
| Lin YC, Dai YT, Hwang SL. The effect of reminiscence on the elderly population: a systematic review. Public Health Nurs 2003; 20(4):297-306. | Not one of included study designs for relevant key question |
| Linn LS, Yager J. The effect of screening, sensitization, and feedback on notation of depression. J Med Educ. 1980;55:942-949. | Does not report included outcomes |
| Lip GYH, Lane DA, Millane TA. Psychological interventions for depression in adolescent and adult congenital heart disease. Cochrane Database of Systematic Reviews 2005;(3). | Not a general primary care population |
| Looper KJ. Potential medical and surgical complications of serotonergic antidepressant medications. *Psychosomatics.* 2007;48:1-9. | Not one of included study design for relevant key question |
| Lowe B, Kroenke K, Grafe K. Detecting and monitoring depression with a two-item questionnaire (PHQ-2). Journal of Psychosomatic Research 2005;58(2):163-71. | Not a screening intervention trial with usual care control group |
| Mackay FR, Dunn NR, Martin RM, Pearce GL, Freemantle SN, Mann RD. Newer antidepressants: a comparison of tolerability in general practice. Br J Gen Pract 1999; 49(448):892-896. | Does not meet design-specific criteria |
| Magruder-Habib K, Zung WW, Feussner JR. Improving physicians' recognition and treatment of depression in general medical care. Results from a randomized clinical trial. Med Care. 1990;28:239-250. | Does not report included outcomes |

| Reference | Reason for exclusion |
|---|---|
| Malt UF, Robak OH, Madsbu HP, Bakke O, Loeb M. The Norwegian naturalistic treatment study of depression in general practice (NORDEP)-I: randomised double blind study. BMJ 1999;318(7192 ):1180 -4. | Non-elderly treatment study |
| Mann AH BR. An evaluation of practice nurses working with general practitioners to treat people with depression. British Journal of General Practice 1998;48(426):875-879. | Not a general primary care population |
| Mastel-Smith BA, McFarlane J, Sierpina M, Malecha A, Haile B. Improving depressive symptoms in community-dwelling older adults: a psychosocial intervention using life review and writing. *J Gerontol Nurs.* 2007;33:13-19. | Not one of included study design for relevant key question |
| McCrone P, Knapp M, Proudfoot J, Ryden C, Cavanagh K, Shapiro DA et al. Cost-effectiveness of computerised cognitive-behavioural therapy for anxiety and depression in primary care: randomised controlled trial. British Journal of Psychiatry 2004;185:55-62. | Non-elderly treatment study |
| McDermut W, Miller IW, Brown RA. The efficacy of group psychotherapy for depression: a meta-analysis and review of the empirical research. Clinical Psychology: Science and Practice 2001; 8(1):98. | Non-elderly treatment study |
| Means-Christensen AJ, Arnau RC, Tonidandel AM, Bramson R, Meagher MW. An efficient method of identifying major depression and panic disorder in primary care. Journal of Behavioral Medicine 2005;28(6):565-72. | Not a screening intervention trial with usual care control group |
| Meijer WE, Heerdink ER, van Eijk JT, Leufkens HG. Adverse events in users of sertraline: results from an observational study in psychiatric practice in The Netherlands. Pharmacoepidemiol Drug Saf 2002; 11(8):655-662. | Comparative-effectiveness |
| Melander H, Ahlqvist-Rastad J, Meijer G, Beermann B. Evidence b(i)ased medicine--selective reporting from studies sponsored by pharmaceutical industry: review of studies in new drug applications. BMJ 2003; 326(7400):1171-1173. | Does not report included outcomes |
| Meyers, Burnett S. Optimizing the use of data generated by geriatric depression treatment studies during a time of diminishing resources. American Journal of Geriatric Psychiatry 15[7], 545-552. 2007. | Not a relevant outcome |
| Milane MS, Suchard MA, Wong ML, Licinio J. Modeling of the temporal patterns of fluoxetine prescriptions and suicide rates in the United States. PLoS Medicine / Public Library of Science 2006; 3(6):e190. | Not one of included study designs for relevant key question |
| Miser WF. Treating depression in older ambulatory patients. J Fam Pract 1998; 47(1):16-17. | Not one of included study designs for relevant key question |
| Mitchell AJ, Subramaniam H. Prognosis of depression in old age compared to middle age: a systematic review of comparative studies. Am J Psychiatry 2005; 162(9):1588-1601. | Comparing subgroups rather than treatment vs. control |

| Reference | Reason for exclusion |
|---|---|
| Moncrieff J, Wessely S, Hardy R. Active placebos versus antidepressants for depression. Cochrane Database of Systematic Reviews 2005;(3):223. | Non-elderly treatment study |
| Moncrieff J, Wessely S, Hardy R. Meta-analysis of trials comparing antidepressants with active placebos. Br J Psychiatry 1998; 172(3):227-231. | Non-elderly treatment study |
| Moore AA, Siu A, Partridge JM, Hays RD, Adams J. A randomized trial of office-based screening for common problems in older persons. American Journal of Medicine 1997;102(4):371-8. | Missing both depression-specific screener and depression-specific outcome |
| Moore JT, Silimperi DR, Bobula JA. Recognition of depression by family medicine residents: the impact of screening. J Fam Pract. 1978;7:509-513. | Does not report included outcomes |
| Moreno RA, Teng CT, Almeida KM, Tavares JH. Hypericum perforatum versus fluoxetine in the treatment of mild to moderate depression: a randomized double-blind trial in a Brazilian sample. Revista Brasileira de Psiquiatria 2006; 28(1):29-32. | Non-elderly treatment study |
| Mottram P, Wilson K, Strobl J. Antidepressants for depressed elderly. Cochrane Database of Systematic Reviews 2006;(1):CD003491. | Focus on treatment comparison, matching, or fine-tuning |
| Mulsan BH SHS. Major depression in older primary care patients conference abstract. 11th Annual Meeting of the American Association for Geriatric Psychiatry 1998; San Diego, California, USA. 8th-11th March,. 1998. | Not one of included study designs for relevant key question |
| Mutch C, Tobin M, Hickie I, Davenport T, Burke D. Improving community-based services for older patients with depression: the benefits of an educational and service initiative. Aust N Z J Psychiatry 2001; 35(4):449-454. | Not one of included study designs for relevant key question |
| Nease DE, Jr., Maloin JM. Depression screening: a practical strategy. Journal of Family Practice 2003;52(2):118-24. | Not a screening intervention trial with usual care control group |
| Nease DE, Klinkman MS, Volk RJ. Improved detection of depression in primary care through severity evaluation. Journal of Family Practice 51(12):1065-70, 2002. | Not a screening intervention trial with usual care control group |
| Nelson JC, Wohlreich MM, Mallinckrodt CH, Detke MJ, Watkin JG, Kennedy JS. Duloxetine for the treatment of major depressive disorder in older patients. Am J Geriatr Psychiatry 2005; 13(3):227-235. | Not one of included study designs for relevant key question |
| Neumeyer-Gromen A, Lampert T, Stark K, Kallischnigg G. Disease management programs for depression: a systematic review and meta-analysis of randomized controlled trials. Med Care 2004; 42(12):1211 | Not a screening intervention trial with usual care control group |
| Newhouse PA, Krishnan KR, Doraiswamy PM, Richter EM, Batzar ED, Clary CM. A double-blind comparison of sertraline and fluoxetine in depressed elderly outpatients. Journal of Clinical Psychiatry 2000;61(8):559-68. | Focus on treatment comparison, matching, or fine-tuning |

| Reference | Reason for exclusion |
| --- | --- |
| Ning J. Observation of the clinical efficacy and safety of mirtazapine on elder depression treatment. *Clnical Pharmaceuticals.* 2004;13:63-64. | Not one of included study design for relevant key question |
| Nunes E, V, Levin FR. Treatment of depression in patients with alcohol or other drug dependence: a meta-analysis. JAMA 2004; 291(15):1887-1896. | Not a general primary care population |
| Nutting PA, Dickinson LM, Rubenstein LV, Keeley RD, Smith JL, Elliott CE. Improving detection of suicidal ideation among depressed patients in primary care. Annals of Family Medicine 2005;3(6):529-36. | Not a screening intervention trial with usual care control group |
| Ong PS. Late-life depression: current issues and new challenges. Ann Acad Med Singapore 2003; 32(6):764-770. | Not one of included study designs for relevant key question |
| Oslin DW THTSJDCW. Probing the safety of medications in the frail elderly: evidence from a randomized clinical trial of sertraline and venlafaxine in depressed nursing home residents. The Journal of clinical psychiatry 2003;(8):875-882. | Focus on treatment comparison, matching, or fine-tuning |
| Oslin DW, Sayers S, Ross J, Kane V, Ten Have T, Conigliaro J et al. Disease management for depression and at-risk drinking via telephone in an older population of veterans. Psychosomatic Medicine 65(6):931 -7, 2003;-Dec. | Comparative-effectiveness |
| Palmer SC, Coyne JC. Screening for depression in medical care: pitfalls, alternatives, and revised priorities. J Psychosom Res 2003; 54(4):279-287. | Not one of included study designs for relevant key question |
| Pampallona S, Bollini P, Tibaldi G, Kupelnick B, Munizza C. Combined pharmacotherapy and psychological treatment for depression: a systematic review. Arch Gen Psychiatry 2004; 61(7):714-719. | Focus on treatment comparison, matching, or fine-tuning |
| Papakostas GI, Petersen T, Denninger JW, Montoya HD, Nierenberg AA, Alpert JE et al. Treatment-related adverse events and outcome in a clinical trial of fluoxetine for major depressive disorder. Ann Clin Psychiatry 2003; 15(3-4):187-192. | Not one of included study designs for relevant key question |
| Patten S, Cipriani A, Brambilla P, Nose M, Barbui C. International dosage differences in fluoxetine clinical trials. Canadian Journal of Psychiatry - Revue Canadienne de Psychiatrie 2005; 50(1):31-38. | Not one of included study designs for relevant key question |
| Pedersen AG. Escitalopram and suicidality in adult depression and anxiety. Int Clin Psychopharmacol 2005; 20(3):139-143. | Updated/covered by another more recent SER/MA |
| Perahia DG, Kajdasz DK, Walker DJ, Raskin J, Tylee A. Duloxetine 60 mg once daily in the treatment of milder major depressive disorder. Int J Clin Pract 2006; 60(5):613-620. | Non-elderly treatment study |

| Reference | Reason for exclusion |
|---|---|
| Pesola GR, Avasarala J. Bupropion seizure proportion among new-onset generalized seizures and drug related seizures presenting to an emergency department. Journal of Emergency Medicine 2002;22(3):235-9. | Not one of included study designs for relevant key question |
| Pignone M, Gaynes B, Lohr K, Rushton JL, Mulrow C. Screening for Depression in Adults. Ann Intern Med 2003; 138(9):767-768. | Used as source document only |
| Pignone MP, Gaynes BN, Rushton JL, Burchell CM, Orleans CT, Mulrow CD et al. Screening for depression in adults: a summary of the evidence for the U.S. Preventive Services Task Force. Ann Intern Med 2002; 136(10):765-776. | Used as source document only |
| Pirraglia PA, Rosen AB, Hermann RC, Olchanski NV, Neumann P. Cost-utility analysis studies of depression management: a systematic review. Am J Psychiatry 2004; 161(12):2155-2162. | Does not report included outcomes |
| Plummer WP. Screening for depression in primary care. Scientific and statistical errors should have been picked up in peer review. BMJ. 2003;326(7396):982. | Not one of included study designs for relevant key question |
| Posternak MA, Miller I. Untreated short-term course of major depression: a meta-analysis of outcomes from studies using wait-list control groups. J Affect Disord 2001; 66(2-3):139-146. | Non-elderly treatment study |
| Proudfoot J, Goldberg D, Mann A, Everitt B, Marks I, Gray JA. Computerized, interactive, multimedia cognitive-behavioural program for anxiety and depression in general practice. Psychological Medicine 2003; 33(2):217-227. | Non-elderly treatment study |
| Proudfoot J, Ryden C, Everitt B, Shapiro DA, Goldberg D, Mann A et al. Clinical efficacy of computerised cognitive-behavioural therapy for anxiety and depression in primary care: randomised controlled trial. British Journal of Psychiatry 2004;185:46-54. | Non-elderly treatment study |
| Rapaport MH, Schneider LS, Dunner DL, Davies JT, Pitts CD. Efficacy of controlled-release paroxetine in the treatment of late-life depression. J Clin Psychiatry 2003; 64(9):1065-1074. | Not one of included study designs for relevant key question |
| Reifler DR, Kessler HS, Bernhard EJ, Leon AC, Martin GJ. Impact of screening for mental health concerns on health service utilization and functional status in primary care patients. Arch Intern Med. 1996;156:2593-2599. | Missing both depression-specific screener and depression-specific outcome |
| Reimherr FW, Strong RE, Marchant BK, Hedges DW, Wender PH. Factors affecting return of symptoms 1 year after treatment in a 62-week controlled study of fluoxetine in major depression. J Clin Psychiatry 2001; 62 Suppl 22:16-23. | Not one of included study designs for relevant key question |

| Reference | Reason for exclusion |
|---|---|
| Reith D, Fountain J, Tilyard M, McDowell R. Antidepressant poisoning deaths in New Zealand for 2001. N Z Med J 2003; 116(1184):U646. | Does not report included outcomes |
| Reynolds CF, III, Dew MA, Pollock BG, Mulsant BH, Frank E, Miller MD et al. Maintenance treatment of major depression in old age. N Engl J Med 2006; 354(11):1130-1138. | Depression prevention or treatment maintenance interventions |
| Reynolds CF, III, Frank E, Dew MA, Houck PR, Miller M, Mazumdar S et al. Treatment of 70(+)-year-olds with recurrent major depression. Excellent short-term but brittle long-term response. American Journal of Geriatric Psychiatry 1999;7(1):64-9. | Depression prevention or treatment maintenance interventions |
| Reynolds CF, III, Frank E, Perel JM, Imber SD, Cornes C, Miller MD et al. Nortriptyline and interpersonal psychotherapy as maintenance therapies for recurrent major depression: a randomized controlled trial in patients older than 59 years. JAMA 1999;281(1):39-45. | Depression prevention or treatment maintenance interventions |
| Reynolds CF, III. Paroxetine treatment of depression in late life. Psychopharmacol Bull 2003; 37:Suppl-34. | Not one of included study designs for relevant key question |
| Richards A, Barkham M, Cahill J, Richards D, Williams C, Heywood P. PHASE: a randomised, controlled trial of supervised self-help cognitive behavioural therapy in primary care. British Journal of General Practice 2003;53(495):764 -70. | Non-elderly treatment study |
| Rihmer Z, Akiskal H. Do antidepressants t(h)reat(en) depressives? Toward a clinically judicious formulation of the antidepressant-suicidality FDA advisory in light of declining national suicide statistics from many countries. J Affect Disord 2006; 94(1-3):3-13. | Not one of included study designs for relevant key question |
| Rokke PD TJJ. Self-management therapy and educational group therapy for depressed elders. Cognitive Therapy & Research 2000;24(1):99-119. | Not one of included study designs for relevant key question |
| Rokke PD, Tomhave JA, Jocic Z. The role of client choice and target selection in self-management therapy for depression in older adults. Psychol Aging 1999; 14(1):155-169. | Not one of included study designs for relevant key question |
| Rollman BL, Hanusa BH, Gilbert T, Lowe HJ, Kapoor WN, Schulberg HC. The electronic medical record. A randomized trial of its impact on primary care physicians' initial management of major depression. Arch Intern Med 2001; 161(2):189-197. | Screen not used in care of patient |
| Rollman BL, Hanusa BH, Lowe HJ, Gilbert T, Kapoor WN, Schulberg HC. A randomized trial using computerized decision support to improve treatment of major depression in primary care. J Gen Intern Med 2002; 17(7):493-503. | Screen not used in care of patient |
| Roose SP, Sackeim HA, Krishnan KR, Pollock BG, Alexopoulos G, Lavretsky H et al. Antidepressant pharmacotherapy in the treatment of depression in the very old: a randomized, placebo-controlled trial. Am J Psychiatry 2004; 161(11):2050-2059. | Not one of included study designs for relevant key question |

| Reference | Reason for exclusion |
|---|---|
| Roose SP, Sackeim HA. Antidepressant medication for the treatment of late-life depression. In: Roose SP, Sackeim HA, eds. Late-life depression. New York, NY: Oxford University Press; 2004:192-202. | Not one of included study designs for relevant key question |
| Roose SP, Schatzberg AF. The Efficacy of Antidepressants in the Treatment of Late-Life Depression. J.Clin.Psychopharmacol. 2005;25(4,Suppl1), S1-S7. | Not one of included study designs for relevant key question |
| Rosenthal MZ, Cheavens JS, Compton JS, Thorp SR, Lynch TR. Thought suppression and treatment outcome in late-life depression. Aging & Mental Health 2005;9(1):35-9. | Focus on treatment comparison, matching, or fine-tuning |
| Rossini D, Serretti A, Franchini L, Mandelli L, Smeraldi E, De RD et al. Sertraline versus fluvoxamine in the treatment of elderly patients with major depression: a double-blind, randomized trial. J Clin Psychopharmacol 2005; 25(5):471-475. | Not one of included study designs for relevant key question |
| Rost K, Pyne JM, Dickinson LM, LoSasso AT. Cost-Effectiveness of Enhancing Primary Care Depression Management on an Ongoing Basis. Annals of Family Medicine 2005; 3(1):7-14. | Does not report included outcomes |
| Sabate E. Depression in Young People and the Elderly. 10-7-2004. World Health Organization. Priority Medicines for Europe and the World. | Not one of included study designs for relevant key question |
| Sauer H, Huppertz-Helmhold S, Dierkes W. Efficacy and safety of venlafaxine ER vs. amitriptyline ER in patients with major depression of moderate severity. Pharmacopsychiatry 2003; 36(5):169-175. | Not one of included study designs for relevant key question |
| Schade CP, Jones ER, Jr., Wittlin BJ. A ten-year review of the validity and clinical utility of depression screening. Psychiatr Serv 1998; 49(1):55-61. | Years covered precede 1999 |
| Schatzberg A, Roose S. A double-blind, placebo-controlled study of venlafaxine and fluoxetine in geriatric outpatients with major depression. Am J Geriatr Psychiatry 2006; 14(4):361-370. | Not one of included study designs for relevant key question |
| Schatzberg AF, Kremer C, Rodrigues HE, Murphy GM, Jr. Double-blind, randomized comparison of mirtazapine and paroxetine in elderly depressed patients. Am J Geriatr Psychiatry 2002; 10(5):541-550. | Focus on treatment comparison, matching, or fine-tuning |
| Schatzberg AF. Efficacy and tolerability of duloxetine, a novel dual reuptake inhibitor, in the treatment of major depressive disorder. J Clin Psychiatry 2003; 64:Suppl-7. | Non-elderly treatment study |
| Schneider LS, Nelson JC, Clary CM, Newhouse P, Krishnan KR, Shiovitz T et al. An 8-week multicenter, parallel-group, double-blind, placebo-controlled study of sertraline in elderly outpatients with major depression. Am J Psychiatry 2003; 160(7):1277-1285. | Not one of included study designs for relevant key question |
| Schoenbaum M, Unutzer J, Sherbourne C, Duan N, Rubenstein LV, Miranda J et al. Cost-effectiveness of practice-initiated quality improvement for depression: results of a randomized controlled trial. JAMA 2001;286(11):1325 -30. | Does not report included outcomes |

| Reference | Reason for exclusion |
|---|---|
| Schone W, Ludwig M. A double-blind study of paroxetine compared with fluoxetine in geriatric patients with major depression. J Clin Psychopharmacol 1993; 13(6 Suppl 2):34S-39S. | Not one of included study designs for relevant key question |
| Schultz CL. The effect of cognitive group therapy in the treatment of depression among residents of senior communities. - Dissertation Abstracts International: Section B: The Sciences and Engineering 1996; 56(9-B):5183. | Not one of included study designs for relevant key question |
| Scogin F, Hamblin D, Beutler L. Bibliotherapy for depressed older adults: a self-help alternative. Gerontologist 1987; 27(3):383-387. | Not one of included study designs for relevant key question |
| Scogin F, Jamison C, Gochneaur K. Comparative efficacy of cognitive and behavioral bibliotherapy for mildly and moderately depressed older adults. J Consult Clin Psychol 1989; 57(3):403-407. | Does not meet quality criteria, including follow-up of less than six weeks |
| Segraves RT, Kavoussi R, Hughes AR, Batey SR, Johnston JA, Donahue R et al. Evaluation of sexual functioning in depressed outpatients: a double-blind comparison of sustained-release bupropion and sertraline treatment. J Clin Psychopharmacol 2000; 20(2):122-128. | Does not report included outcomes |
| Serby M, Yu M. Overview: depression in the elderly. Mt Sinai J Med 2003; 70(1):38-44. | Not one of included study designs for relevant key question |
| Sheffield RE, Lo Sasso AT, Young CH, Way K. Selective serotonin reuptake inhibitor usage patterns as risk factors for hospitalization. Administration & Policy in Mental Health 2002; 30(2):121-139. | Does not report included outcomes |
| Sheikh JI, Cassidy EL, Doraiswamy PM, Salomon RM, Hornig M, Holland PJ et al. Efficacy, safety, and tolerability of sertraline in patients with late-life depression and comorbid medical illness. J Am Geriatr Soc 2004; 52(1):86-92. | Not one of included study designs for relevant key question |
| Simon GE, VonKorff M, Heiligenstein JH, Revicki DA, Grothaus L, Katon W et al. Initial antidepressant choice in primary care. Effectiveness and cost of fluoxetine vs tricyclic antidepressants. JAMA 1996; 275(24):1897-1902. | Non-elderly treatment study |
| Simpson S, Corney R, Fitzgerald P, Beecham J. A randomized controlled trial to evaluate the effectiveness and cost-effectiveness of psychodynamic counselling for general practice patients with chronic depression. Psychol Med 2003; 33(2):229-239. | Non-elderly treatment study, comparative-effectiveness |
| Sirey JA, Bruce ML, Alexopoulos GS. The Treatment Initiation Program: an intervention to improve depression outcomes in older adults. American Journal of Psychiatry 2005;162(1):184-6. | Focus on treatment comparison, matching, or fine-tuning |
| Sloane RB SFSL. Interpersonal therapy vs. nortriptyline for depression in the elderly. Clinical and pharmacological studies in psychiatric disorders Biological psychiatry - new prospects 344-6p 1985. | Not one of included study designs for relevant key question |

| Reference | Reason for exclusion |
|---|---|
| Smit F, Ederveen A, Cuijpers P, Deeg D, Beekman A. Opportunities for cost-effective prevention of late-life depression: an epidemiological approach. Arch Gen Psychiatry 2006; 63(3):290-296. | Not a screening intervention trial with usual care control group |
| Sondergard L, Kvist K, Lopez AG, Andersen PK, Kessing LV. Temporal changes in suicide rates for persons treated and not treated with antidepressants in Denmark during 1995-1999. Acta Psychiatr.Scand. 2006; 114 (3):168-176. | Information included in Sondergard Int Clin Psychopharmacol 2006 |
| Steed L, Cooke D, Newman S. A systematic review of psychosocial outcomes following education, self-management and psychological interventions in diabetes mellitus. Patient Educ Couns 2003; 51(1):5 | Not a general primary care population |
| Stimpson N, Agrawal N, Lewis G. Randomised controlled trials investigating pharmacological and psychological interventions for treatment-refractory depression. Br J Psychiatry 2002; 181(4):284-294. | Not a general primary care population |
| Storosum JG, Elferink AJ, van Zwieten BJ, van den Brink W, Gersons BP, van Strik R et al. Short-term efficacy of tricyclic antidepressants revisited: a meta-analytic study. Eur Neuropsychopharmacol 2001;11(2):173-180. | Non-elderly treatment study |
| Suh T, Gallo JJ. Symptom profiles of depression among general medical service users compared with specialty mental health service users. Psychol Med 1997; 27(5):1051-1063. | Does not report included outcomes |
| Swindle RW, Rao JK, Helmy A, Plue L, Zhou XH, Eckert GJ et al. Integrating clinical nurse specialists into the treatment of primary care patients with depression. Int J Psychiatry Med 2003; 33(1):17-37. | Focus on treatment comparison, matching, or fine-tuning |
| Taylor WD, Doraiswamy PM. A systematic review of antidepressant placebo-controlled trials for geriatric depression: limitations of current data and directions for the future. Neuropsychopharmacology 2004; 29(12):2285 | Updated/covered by another more recent SER/MA |
| Thase ME. Effects of venlafaxine on blood pressure: a meta-analysis of original data from 3744 depressed patients. J Clin Psychiatry 1998; 59(10):502-508. | Does not report included outcomes |
| Thomas HV, Lewis G, Watson M, Bell T, Lyons I, Lloyd K et al. Computerised patient-specific guidelines for management of common mental disorders in primary care: a randomised controlled trial. British Journal of General Practice 2004;54(508):832-7. | Focus on treatment comparison, matching, or fine-tuning |
| Thomas SP. From The Editor--Caution Urged in Prescribing Psychotropic Drugs for Older Patients. Issues Ment.Health Nurs. 2005;26(4), 357-358. | Not one of included study designs for relevant key question |
| Thompson C, Kinmonth AL, Stevens L, Peveler RC, Stevens A, Ostler KJ et al. Effects of a clinical-practice guideline and practice-based education on detection and outcome of depression in primary care: Hampshire Depression Project randomised controlled trial. Lancet 355(9199):185-91, 2000. | Screen not used in care of patient |

| Reference | Reason for exclusion |
|---|---|
| Thompson LW, Gallagher D, Breckenridge JS. Comparative effectiveness of psychotherapies for depressed elders. J Consult Clin Psychol 1987; 55(3):385-390. | Not one of included study designs for relevant key question |
| Townsend E, Hawton K, Altman DG, Arensman E, Gunnell D, Hazell P et al. The efficacy of problem-solving treatments after deliberate self-harm: meta-analysis of randomized controlled trials with respect to depression, hopelessness and improvement in problems. Psychol Med 2001; 31(6):979-988. | Non-elderly treatment study |
| Trindade E, Menon D, Topfer LA, Coloma C. Adverse effects associated with selective serotonin reuptake inhibitors and tricyclic antidepressants: a meta-analysis. Can Med Assoc J 1998; 159(10):1245-1252. | Years covered precede 1999 |
| University of York. NHS Centre for Reviews and Dissemination. Improving the recognition and management of depression in primary care. Eff Health Care 2002;7(5):1-12. | Not one of included study designs for relevant key question |
| Unutzer J, Katon W, Callahan CM, Williams JW, Jr., Hunkeler E, Harpole L et al. Collaborative care management of late-life depression in the primary care setting: a randomized controlled trial. JAMA 2002; 288(22):2836-2845. | Focus on treatment comparison, matching, or fine-tuning |
| van de Meent H, Geurts AC, van Limbeek J. Pharmacologic treatment of poststroke depression: a systematic review of the literature. Topics in Stroke Rehabilitation 2003;10(1):79-92. | Not a general primary care population |
| van den Berg S, Shapiro DA, Bickerstaffe D, Cavanagh K. Computerized cognitive-behaviour therapy for anxiety and depression: a practical solution to the shortage of trained therapists. Journal of Psychiatric & Mental Health Nursing 2004;11(5):508-13. | Not a treatment outcomes study |
| van Os TW, van den Brink RH, Tiemens BG, Jenner JA, van der Meer K, Ormel J. Are effects of depression management training for General Practitioners on patient outcomes mediated by improvements in the process of care? J Affect Disord 2004;80(2-3):173-179. | Not a screening intervention trial with usual care control group |
| van Walraven C, Mamdani MM, Wells PS, Williams JI. Inhibition of serotonin reuptake by antidepressants and upper gastrointestinal bleeding in elderly patients: retrospective cohort study. BMJ 2001;323(7314):655-658. | Updated/covered by another more recent SER/MA |
| Verkaik R, van Weert JC, Francke AL. The effects of psychosocial methods on depressed, aggressive and apathetic behaviors of people with dementia: a systematic review. Int J Geriatr Psychiatry 2005; 20(4):301-314. | Not a general primary care population |

| Reference | Reason for exclusion |
|---|---|
| Viney LL, Benjamin YN, Preston CA. An evaluation of personal construct therapy for the elderly. Br J Med Psychol 1989; 62(Pt 1):35-41. | Not one of included study designs for relevant key question |
| Volkers AC, Nuyen J, Verhaak PF, Schellevis FG. The problem of diagnosing major depression in elderly primary care patients. Journal of Affective Disorders 2004;82(2):259-63. | Not one of included study designs for relevant key question |
| Von Korff M, Goldberg D. Improving outcomes in depression. BMJ 2001; 323(7319):948-949. | Not one of included study designs for relevant key question |
| Vos T, Haby MM, Barendregt JJ, Kruijshaar M, Corry J, Andrews G. The burden of major depression avoidable by longer-term treatment strategies. Arch Gen Psychiatry 2004; 61(11):1097-1103. | Does not report included outcomes |
| Wagner W, Zaborny BA, Gray TE. Fluvoxamine. A review of its safety profile in world-wide studies. Int Clin Psychopharmacol 1994; 9(4):223-227. | Updated/covered by another more recent SER/MA |
| Walsh BT, Sysko R. Placebo control groups in trials of major depressive disorder among older patients. J Clin Psychopharmacol 2005; 25(4:Suppl 1):Suppl-33. | Focus on interventions that are not primarily CBT-related or IPT in nature |
| Walsh MT, Dinan TG. Selective serotonin reuptake inhibitors and violence: a review of the available evidence. Acta Psychiatr Scand 2001; 104(2):84-91. | Updated/covered by another more recent SER/MA |
| Watson LC, Pignone MP. Screening accuracy for late-life depression in primary care: a systematic review. J Fam Pract 2003; 52(12):956-964. | Not a screening intervention trial with usual care control group |
| Weatherall M. A randomized controlled trial of the Geriatric Depression Scale in an inpatient ward for older adults. Clin Rehabil. 2000;14:186-191. | Does not report included outcomes |
| Weihs KL, Settle EC, Jr., Batey SR, Houser TL, Donahue RM, Ascher JA. Bupropion sustained release versus paroxetine for the treatment of depression in the elderly. J Clin Psychiatry 2000; 61(3):196-202. | Comparative-effectiveness |
| Weinrieb RM, Auriacombe M, Lynch KG, Chang KM, Lewis JD. A critical review of selective serotonin reuptake inhibitor-associated bleeding: balancing the risk of treating hepatitis C-infected patients. J Clin Psychiatry 2003; 64(12):1502 | Not a general primary care population |
| Wells JL, Seabrook JA, Stolee P, Borrie MJ, Knoefel F. State of the art in geriatric rehabilitation. Part II: clinical challenges. Arch Phys Med Rehabil 2003; 84(6):898-903. | Not a general primary care population |
| Wen SW, Walker M. Risk of fetal exposure to tricyclic antidepressants. J Obstet Gynaecol Can 2004; 26(10):887-892. | Focus on pregnancy-related screening |
| Wessely S, Kerwin R. Suicide Risk and the SSRIs. JAMA: Journal of the American Medical Association 2004;292(3), 379-381. | Not one of included study designs for relevant key question |

| Reference | Reason for exclusion |
|---|---|
| Wessinger S, Kaplan M, Choi L et al. Increased use of selective serotonin reuptake inhibitors in patients admitted with gastrointestinal haemorrhage: a multicentre retrospective analysis. *Aliment Pharmacol Ther.* 2006;23:937-944. | Not a primary care population |
| Westen D, Morrison K. A multidimensional meta-analysis of treatments for depression, panic, and generalized anxiety disorder: an empirical examination of the status of empirically supported therapies. J Consult Clin Psychol 2001; 69(6):875-899. | Non-elderly treatment study |
| Whitehead C, Moss S, Cardno A, Lewis G. Antidepressants for people with both schizophrenia and depression. Cochrane Database of Systematic Reviews 2005;(3). | Not a general primary care population |
| Whittington CJ, Kendall T, Fonagy P, Cottrell D, Cotgrove A, Boddington E. Selective serotonin reuptake inhibitors in childhood depression: systematic review of published versus unpublished data. Lancet 2004; 363(9418):1341-1345. | Focus on children or adolescents |
| Whyte EM, Mulsant BH. Post stroke depression: epidemiology, pathophysiology, and biological treatment. Biol Psychiatry 2002; 52(3):253-264. | Not a general primary care population |
| Wilson KCM, Mottram PG. Long-term treatments for older depressed people. Cochrane Database of Systematic Reviews 2005;(3). | Depression prevention or treatment maintenance intervention |
| Wisner KL, Gelenberg AJ, Leonard H, Zarin D, Frank E. Pharmacologic treatment of depression during pregnancy. JAMA 1999; 282(13):1264-1269. | Focus on pregnancy-related screening |
| Wohlfarth T, Storosum JG, Elferink AJ, van Zwieten BJ, Fouwels A, van den BW. Response to tricyclic antidepressants: independent of gender? Am J Psychiatry 2004; 161(2):370-372. | Non-elderly treatment study |
| Wright JH, Wright AS, Albano AM, Basco MR, Goldsmith LJ, Raffield T et al. Computer-assisted cognitive therapy for depression: maintaining efficacy while reducing therapist time. American Journal of Psychiatry 2005;162(6):1158 -64. | Non-elderly treatment study |
| Zetin M. Psychopharmaco-hazardology: major hazards of treating depression and anxiety. Comprehensive Therapy 2004;30(1):18-24. | Not one of included study designs for relevant key question |
| Zung WW, Magill M, Moore JT, George DT. Recognition and treatment of depression in a family medicine practice. J Clin Psychiatry. 1983;44:3-6. | Does not meet quality criteria |

**Appendix G. Table 8. Fair- to poor-quality cohort study details.**

**Gibbons 2007:**[146] A fair-to-poor quality observational study of Veteran's Administration patients identified 226,866 patients with evidence of depression in 2003 or 2004, and no history of treatment for depression in the previous 3 years. Use of SSRIs, non-SSRI second generation agents (bupropion, mirtazapine, nefazodone, and venlafaxine), and TCAs was abstracted from electronic medical records. Among these patients, 114,475 were treated with a single type of antidepressants (SSRI, other second generation, or TCA), 52,959 were treated with antidepressants in more than one of these categories, and 59,432 had no record of antidepressant use. Suicide attempts (including those that were fatal) which led to contact with the VA system over 6-24 months after new antidepressant treatment initiation were identified using diagnosis codes in the medical record. The study was not able to examine all suicide-related deaths. The overall rate of suicide attempts in those initiating SSRI treatment (alone or in combination with other medications) was 36.4/10,000 compared with 33.5/10,000 suicide attempts among those diagnosed but not treated. The remaining analyses are not useful since they compared the experience of a selected subgroup who received only one type of antidepressant, which excluded 26 percent of all depressed patients (and 34 percent of those treated with antidepressants). Further, comparisons between medications for this subgroup are likely confounded by indication, since more patients with major depressive disorder were treated with non-SSRIs than with SSRIs.

**Sondergard 2006:**[144] In a fair-to-poor quality cohort study using national registries for all Danish prescriptions and deaths in 1995-1999, Sondergard and colleagues determined the rates of suicides per 10,000 person-years in 438,625 adults dispensed any type of antidepressants (24 different medications) for any indication over up to five years of follow-up.[144] Mean follow-up was not reported. Suicides in persons treated with antidepressants ranged from 11.5 to 48.6 per 10,000 person-years, with rates in men two-three times higher than those in women. Seventy percent of the 1474 persons receiving antidepressants who committed suicide did so during the first month of treatment. In the untreated control group that was selected "randomly" from all non-users, there were 1.3 suicides per 10,000 person-years of follow-up (2.0 in men and 0.56 in women). More precise estimates of suicide rates in antidepressant-treated adults are not available as all rates of suicides were reported only by drug type and numbers of dispenses, and this data has a high potential for confounding by indication (particularly since patients being treated for all indications were examined). Confounding by indication is also a concern since these were not clearly incident users, as prior treatment history was not considered (except for excluding those with previous lithium dispenses). Comparisons of the untreated controls with the treated patients is further limited by lack of matching or adjustment for potential confounders such as age.

**Mackay 1999:**[143,145] Two fair-to-poor quality studies reported survey data examining GP-reports of suicide and other adverse events in patients identified using Prescription Event Monitoring Database records from 1987-1996.[143,145] Investigators surveyed GPs six months after one of their patients received their first prescription during the post-marketing period for one of seven newly approved antidepressants (4 SSRIs two other second-generation antidepressants, one first-generation). Recall surveys focused on indications, starting and stopping dates, response to treatment, events during and after treatment (defined to elicit possible-drug related events), and reasons for discontinuation. Response rates were low (55 to 64 percent). There were at least 10,000 persons in the final cohort for each antidepressant, and at least 71 to 80 percent of the patients were being treated for depression, excluding any patients treated for mania, hypomania, agitation, or anxiety. The combined rate for suicide and "parasuicide" (not further defined) among those taking any of the antidepressant drugs was 324-672/10,000 person-years, depending on medication. Data were not reported on the completeness of returned surveys or on whether doctors used medical records or simply recall in completing forms. Given the low GP response rates, estimates could be too high if doctors preferentially reported on patients with serious side-effects or too low if the opposite were true.

**Appendix G. Table 9. FDA summary.**

In the 2006 FDA report, there was a large difference in event rates for suicide, particularly in patients with MDD, and in suicidal behaviors, compared with the findings in multiple other independent analyses. Particularly puzzling is the difference in event rates between the 2006 report and another 2006 publication representing similar FDA work apparently using some of the same datasets. The 2006 FDA report provides several explanations for its lower event rates than earlier reports by Gunnell and Fergusson, including potential over-counting of multiple suicide-related events per person in these other analyses. However, since suicide cannot be counted twice, this does not explain the two- to four- fold reduction in suicide rates in the 2006 FDA report compared to others evaluating similar patient groups. Other possible explanations are: 1) differences in event definitions (definitions for suicide-related behaviors may have excluded events counted elsewhere;[138] 2) differences in event determination (it is not clear the FDA searched for adverse events in case record forms to identify events not flagged as drug-related or significant by the trial investigator as did the MHRA-related work);[105] and 3) differences in event categorization, including the fact that the FDA relied on companies to categorize adverse events using a protocol (as did the MHRA) and required narratives for all potential suicide-related adverse effects, but did not collect or review them all (in contrast to the requirements in the MHRA-related analyses). Potential differences due to event categorization could not be assessed since the FDA report did not provide event numbers for serious adverse events that were not included in the suicide-related outcomes (i.e., self-injurious behavior, intent unknown, not enough information-fatal, not enough information-non-fatal) and did not provide the numbers upon request. Finally, 4) a lower event rate in the FDA report could reflect the time frame in which adverse events could be counted. This limited the FDA report to active treatment only, and events were not counted if they occurred during placebo run-in before randomization (which is appropriate) or greater than one day after medication discontinuation (which could lead to underascertainment, particularly with so many discontinuing treatment early). In one of the observational studies we reviewed in which 69 suicides occurred in adults after receiving their first dispense of antidepressants, the person was not taking antidepressants at the time of their suicide in about half of the cases (52 percent).[128]

The FDA indicated it requests information on any death occurring within the period ending 90 days after the intended treatment period in order to look for informative censoring. However, it is not clear if or how this reporting approach affected the final analyses. In considering differences between its 2006 report and others, the FDA rightly notes that it has a superior method with individual level meta-analysis as compared to trial level meta-analysis. However, the differences between the FDA 2006 report findings and other meta-analyses would not be primarily explained by these analytic differences. Finally, by choosing a primary outcome that combined ideation with behavior, we found that many of the FDA report's results were not clarifying. Raw event data from the 2006 FDA report indicate that the impact of antidepressants, compared with placebo, on suicidal behaviors differs in direction from the impact on suicidal ideation. These findings are corroborated in other reviews that find a statistically significant impact on suicidal behavior, but not ideation, in the few patient subgroups with any suicide-related adverse events.

CPSIA information can be obtained
at www.ICGtesting.com
Printed in the USA
LVHW012134270422
717384LV00007B/427